THE ART OF MEDICINE IN EARLY CHINA

In this book, Miranda Brown investigates the myths that acupuncturists and herbalists have told about the birth of the healing arts. Moving from the Han (206 BC–AD 220) and Song (960–1279) dynasties to the twentieth century, Brown traces the rich history of Chinese medical historiography and the gradual emergence of the archive of medical tradition. She exposes the historical circumstances that shaped the current image of medical progenitors: the ancient bibliographers, medieval editors, and modern reformers and defenders of Chinese medicine who contributed to the contemporary shape of the archive. Brown demonstrates how ancient and medieval ways of knowing live on in popular narratives of medical history, both in modern Asia and in the West. She also reveals the surprising and often unacknowledged debt that contemporary scholars owe to their premodern forbearers for the categories, frameworks, and analytic tools with which to study the distant past.

Miranda Brown is an associate professor of Asian languages and cultures at the University of Michigan. She has published numerous articles on various aspects of Chinese medical and cultural history in both English and Chinese. She is the author of *The Politics of Mourning in Early China* (2007) and the coauthor of *A Brief History of Chinese Civilization* (2012, with Conrad Schirokauer). She is a coeditor of *Fragments: Interdisciplinary Approaches to the Study of Ancient and Medieval Pasts*, a journal that she founded with leading U.S. scholars.

THE ART OF MEDICINE IN EARLY CHINA

THE ANCIENT AND MEDIEVAL ORIGINS OF A MODERN ARCHIVE

MIRANDA BROWN
University of Michigan

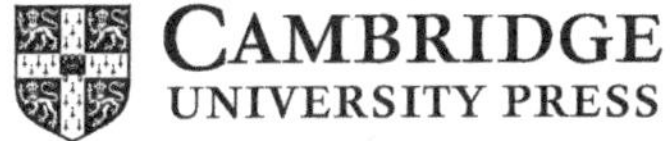

CAMBRIDGE
UNIVERSITY PRESS

32 Avenue of the Americas, New York, NY 10013-2473, USA

Cambridge University Press is part of the University of Cambridge.

It furthers the University's mission by disseminating knowledge in the pursuit of education, learning, and research at the highest international levels of excellence.

www.cambridge.org
Information on this title: www.cambridge.org/9781107097056

First published 2015

Printed in the United States of America

A catalog record for this publication is available from the British Library.

Library of Congress Cataloging in Publication Data
Brown, Miranda, 1975–, author.
The art of medicine in early China : the ancient and medieval origins of a modern archive / Miranda Brown.
p. ; cm.
Chapter 1 of this book was originally published in Medical History, volume 56, no. 3 (2012). Chapter 4 of this book was originally published in Chang'an 26 BCE : From Dreams to Ditches (Seattle: University of Washington Press, 2015).
Includes bibliographical references and index.
ISBN 978-1-107-09705-6 (hbk.)
I. Medical history. II. Chang'an 26 BCE. III. Title.
[DNLM: 1. Medicine in Literature – China. 2. Medicine, Chinese Traditional – history – China. 3. Physicians – China – Biography. 4. History, Ancient – China. 5. History, Medieval – China. WZ 70 JC6]
R604.A1
610.92'251–dc23 2014045601

ISBN 978-1-107-09705-6 Hardback

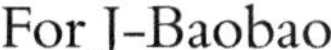

For J-Baobao

Chapter 1 of this book was originally published as "Who Was He? Reflections on China's First Medical 'Naturalist,'" *Med. Hist.* 56.3 (2012): 366–89. Reproduced with permission from Cambridge University Press.

Chapter 4 of this book was originally published as "Looking Backward: Explaining the Rise of a Medical Tradition in Han China." In Griet VanKeerberghen and Michael Nylan eds., *Chang'an 26 BCE: An Augustan Age in China* (Seattle: University of Washington Press, 2015). Reproduced with permission from University of Washington Press.

TABLE OF CONTENTS

ILLUSTRATIONS

TABLES

ACKNOWLEDGMENTS

Some ten years ago, I set out to write a book about medicine in early China. The book is overdue, because of the predictable turns of academic life after tenure. But the book's belated arrival also owes something to happier turns of events. In the process of founding a journal with my colleagues at the University of Michigan and elsewhere, *Fragments: Interdisciplinary Approaches to the Study of Ancient and Medieval Pasts*, I discovered a new community and sense of camaraderie among scholars of the premodern. It is my hope that this sense of community – and our shared conviction that the ancient and medieval worlds remain relevant in the present – informs this book's design.

Over the last decade, I have indebted myself to many parties: grant-giving organizations, colleagues, editors, and friends. Two grants made the early research for this project possible: the Chiang Ching-Kuo Foundation and the National Endowment for the Humanities (Ref. FA 52204–06). In addition, I inflicted draft chapters on scores of graduate classmates, colleagues, former students, and friends: Bridie Andrews, Robert Campany, Ardeta Gjikola, Kevin Landdeck, Joshua MacDonald, Liu Yan, Pablo Mercado, Griet VanKeerberghen, Yi-Li Wu, Nicholas Tackett, Thomas Trautmann, and Vivian Nutton (who read an early draft of Chapter 1 and sent back encouraging feedback as the editor of *Medical History*). This project also benefitted from discussions with Micah Auerback, Saul Allen, and Nancy Florida.

In addition, I would like to thank Michael Nylan (my teacher) and Nathan Sivin (Michael's teacher). Michael did more than offer her constructive criticisms of an earlier version of Chapter 4, a *decade* after I finished graduate school. She also offered me her friendship during a trying period of my life. For his part, Nathan perused what are now Chapters 3 and 5, proffering some perspicacious observations that pushed my book in its current direction.

Three colleagues deserve medals – for their endurance. For four long years, David Spafford and Charles Sanft trekked through every draft chapter that I produced. They pondered the same passages multiple times, corrected translations and transcriptions, offered advice about argumentation and style, and lent me their ear as the revisions spun out of control. For his part, Bill Baxter dug into the entire manuscript when it was least coherent and then read successive drafts of the introduction in the months to come. Without his input, I doubt that this book would have ever been finished.

Cambridge University Press also deserves special mention for the handling of this manuscript: Beatrice Rehl for taking on this project in the first place and being patient as I struggled to locate a narrative thread; Asya Graf for making the review process a smooth one and e-mail pleasurable again; and Marc Anderson for talking me through the entire permissions process and answering my questions on weekends. I would also like to thank the two reviewers commissioned by the press for their candid and timely comments.

My students at the University of Michigan also played their part in making this book. I vetted introductions, translations, and chapters to successive cohorts of my Chinese medicine class. Sherley Wetherhold, a current undergraduate and a gifted writer, edited the manuscript with efficiency and grace. Finally, a special word of thanks goes to one class in particular (Fall 2013). Just as my morale and energy fell to all new lows, my students, fledgling hedge fund managers and physicians in training, pleasantly surprised me. Twice a week for a term, they argued about ancient sex manuals, pointed out Galen's violation of HIPAA regulations, and analyzed the toxins in ancient preparations. Their boisterousness saved me loads of money on ginseng. It also reminded me why I was writing my book in the first place (namely, that doing ancient history is *fun*).

Finally, a word of appreciation for J-Baobao, my husband and best friend. He not only read every word of the book (out loud) but also tasted the meds. While I can't promise that the next book will be any easier to write, I am hoping that he will find the next subject to be tastier!

CHRONOLOGY

Zhou dynasty	**1045–221 BC**
Spring and Autumn	771–453 BC
Warring States	453–221 BC
Qin dynasty	**221–206 BC**
Han dynasty	**206 BC–AD 220**
Western Han	206 BC–AD 9
Xin dynasty (or Wang Mang interregnum)	9–23
Eastern Han	25–220
Six Dynasties period	**220–581**
Three Kingdoms	220–65
Jin dynasty	265–420
Western Jin	265–316
Eastern Jin	317–420
Northern and Southern dynasties	**385–589**
Northern dynasties	420–589
Southern dynasties	386–534
Sui dynasty	**581–618**
Tang dynasty	**618–907**
Five Dynasties period	**907–60**

Song dynasty	**960–1279**
Northern Song	960–1127
Southern Song	1127–1279
Jin (Jurchen) dynasty	**1115–1234**
Yuan (Mongol) dynasty	**1271–1368**
Ming dynasty	**1368–1644**
Qing (Manchu) dynasty	**1644–1911**
Republic of China	**1912–1949**
People's Republic of China	**1949–**

AUTHOR'S NOTE ON TRANSLATIONS AND CHINESE TEXT

All translations are my own unless otherwise noted.

When possible, Chinese text is transcribed as it appears in the original edition. When I have substituted a character for the nonstandard graph that appears in the original text, the substitution is placed in parentheses (). When the character cannot be transcribed, or cannot be transcribed as a standard character, the notation [?] appears. Finally, the notation [...] is used to indicate a lacuna in the text.

INTRODUCTION

THIS BOOK BEGAN AS AN INDICTMENT OF THE PRESENT. My goal was to expose and clear away the distortions introduced by modern ideologies into our interpretation of ancient Chinese medical history beginning in the nineteenth century. I had expected to find evidence of these ideologies in the various retellings of ancient medical history – namely, narratives that assume the progress of knowledge over the ages and relate the triumph of reason over superstition. This, of course, I found. But to my surprise, there was more. In modern retellings of Chinese medical history, I also discovered the tenacious survival of ancient historiographical practices, traces of which are everywhere, expressed in the selection and interpretation of the archive.

I first became aware of old historiographical practices while looking for evidence of modern bias. Nowhere did such bias seem more obvious than in the presentation of ancient figures by twentieth-century historians. Take Joseph Needham (1900–95) and Lu Gwei-djen 魯桂珍 (1904–91), for instance, two individuals often referred to as pioneers in the history of Chinese science. Their views on the origins of Chinese medicine are set forth in two seminal works, *Celestial Lancets: A History and Rationale of Acupuncture and Moxa* (1980) and an influential volume on medicine in *Science and Civilisation* (2000). Their story about the progress of Chinese medicine enumerated the achievements of what they called the "fathers of medicine."

Chinese medical history begins with the "liberation" of healing practices from the older, purely magico-religious understandings of illness. According to Needham and Lu, the signs of such a shift may be glimpsed in the prognoses of Attendant He 和 (fl. 541 BC), whose "lectures" revealed the advance from magic and religion to primitive scientific theory.[1] Attendant He's breakthrough was then followed by the achievements of Bian Que 扁鵲, a mythical court physician with murky dates and lauded as a Chinese "Hippocrates." Next in the sequence of medical progenitors was Chunyu Yi 淳于意 (fl. ca. 180–154 BC) of the Han 漢 dynasty (206 BC–AD 220), whose records of consultation proved that "the examination of the sick person, the investigation of the clinical history, the comparison of data from different examinations, and the therapeutic deductions all formed part of a discipline which constituted a valid and valuable precursor of contemporary clinical science."[2] The achievements of Zhang Ji 張機 in the early third century AD were next, as Zhang was the "first to set forth prescriptions in detail, and the first to classify febrile illnesses. . . ."[3] Then came Hua Tuo 華佗 (d. AD 208), who won "enduring fame for his skill in surgery and related disciplines, his early use of some kind of anesthesia, and his discoveries and inventions of medical gymnastics. . . ."[4] Last were two figures of late antiquity, Huangfu Mi 皇甫謐 (AD 215–282) and Wang Xi 王熙 (AD 180–270?): the first purportedly composed the earliest work on acupuncture, whereas the other perfected the techniques of pulse diagnosis.[5]

Needham and Lu surely were not alone in imbuing ancient healers with modern significance. Similar descriptions run throughout the literature, a literature Nathan Sivin criticizes for "chronicling the careers of Great Men."[6] Indeed, a scan of the historiography reveals a similar emphasis on the ancient healer's achievements. Notably, such an emphasis is found in the *History of Chinese Medicine* (*Zhongguo yixue shi* 中國醫學史) by Chen Bangxian 陳邦賢 (1889–1976), initially published in 1919 and sometimes described as the first modern history of Chinese medicine. The same historiographical tendency is also on display in an important work by Fan Xingzhun 范行準 (1906–98), a *Short History of Chinese Medicine* (*Zhongguo yixue shilüe* 中國醫學史略; 1986). There, Fan included many of the same descriptions of Needham's "fathers of medicine": Attendant He's famous discussion of illness, Bian Que's innovations in diagnosis and therapy, Chunyu Yi's clinical case histories, Zhang Ji's painstaking emphasis on empirical observation, Hua Tuo's surgical feats, and the treatises by Huangfu Mi and Wang Xi.[7]

Over time, what I found most striking about the medical fathers was not so much their modern significance as their sheer ubiquity. They appear throughout the current scholarship, which has achieved considerable sophistication since Needham and can hardly be thought of as hagiography. Consider the case of mythical Bian Que; scholars like Yamada Keiji 山田慶兒 no longer write about Bian Que as a historical personage.[8] Nevertheless, scholars continue to use Bian Que's biography in a dynastic history as a source, culling it for clues about ancient medical theory and for hints of professional conflict between healers and their occult competitors. Similarly, current historians have moved far beyond Needham's naïve reading of the textual record, and they no longer treat Chunyu Yi's biography as evidence of an "advanced clinical science." Even so, the biography continues to supply scholars with the materials to reconstruct practices of transmission, to examine medical theory in the second century BC, and to nuance our understandings of the relationship between medicine and divination.[9]

The relevance of the ancient medical fathers to contemporary scholarship is perhaps clearest in a recent work by Liao Yuqun 廖育群, *Traditional Chinese Medicine* (2011). Like other contemporary historians, Liao approaches his sources with an admirable judiciousness and a broad knowledge of the archaeological record. Still, Liao finds it difficult to write Chinese medical history without invoking the words and deeds attributed to the ancient progenitors of the craft. This is evident from a short chapter entitled "Stories about Famous Doctors in History," which contains descriptions of the ancient progenitors and references many of the same stories used by Needham and countless others.[10]

The medical fathers' iron grip on the historical imagination is further evident in popular presentations of Chinese medicine. We find them in illustrated cartoons that depict scenes from the life of Bian Que, storybook versions of Chinese medicine from the People's Republic of China, and popular websites about Chinese medicine targeted at Americans seeking alternative therapies. All of these describe the achievements of the ancient medical fathers, and some paint portraits of them. For example, the National Institutes of Health sponsored a digital website that summarized an exhibit held at the National Library of Medicine from October 1999 to May 2000. We find there the history of Chinese medicine recounted through the descriptions of legendary and historical innovators: the Yellow Emperor, the Divine Husbandman, Zhang Ji, and so forth; such descriptions were also accompanied by portraits of the ancestors (see Figure 1).[11]

Where did these fathers of medicine come from? And how did these figures acquire such a prominent place in both the modern historiography and popular imagination? The questions deserve to be asked because the medical fathers hardly represented a natural grouping. After all, the figures were very different from one another. Some of them, particularly Bian Que, depicted in early stone reliefs as half-man and half-bird,

載名亞聖
論證表裏虛實
漢張仲景傷寒
張仲景
華元化
魏有華
佗設立
瘡科
剮骨療
疾神效
巧多

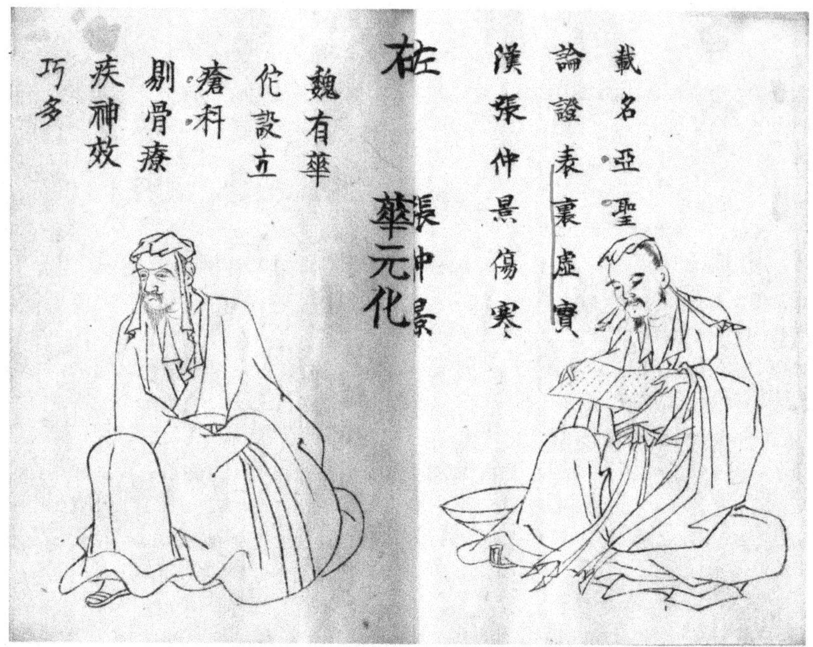

Figure 1 A page from *Illustrations and Eulogies for Healers and Transcendents* (*Yi xian tuzan* 醫僊圖讃; 1599), included in the National Institutes of Health exhibit for Chinese medical history. The right displays a portrait of Zhang Ji and the left of Hua Tuo. The inscription from left to right reads: "He carries the reputation of a secondary sage. He classified the signs with respect to the inside and outside [of the body], as well as the emptiness and fullness [of the pulse]. Zhang Zhongjing [i.e., Zhang Ji] of the Han, [with the] *Treatise on Cold Damage Disorders*. In the Wei dynasty, there was Hua Tuo, who established the specialty of [diagnosing and treating] external harm. He separated the flesh from bones and cured the illnesses [of the body]."

were clearly mythical beings. Others, such as Chunyu Yi and Zhang Ji, had a distinctly mundane feel to them. More importantly, the sources that Needham and other historians used to explain the contributions of these figures – and thus to construct a broader narrative of healing in ancient China – were hardly obvious candidates for medical history. Such sources were materials of disparate periods, authors, audiences, and aims. Very few of them in fact were actually medical treatises, being composed of bits and pieces of historical chronicles, dynastic histories – and worse still, political allegories.[12] Given such diversity, how did these figures and pieces of text ever find their way into a single narrative? In other words, what principles or circumstances conspired to give them their stubborn place within the archive?

In raising these questions, my objective is not to criticize the medical fathers as a modern anachronism. On the contrary, this book will show that the fathers *do* have their place in Chinese medical history (although their significance is quite different from what Needham imagined). To get somewhat ahead of myself, I will argue that the medical fathers are less useful for explaining the development of Chinese medical practice or theory in antiquity. Instead, they are of interest because they reveal how early Chinese authors provided modern historians like Needham not only with the raw materials, but also the categories, genres, and objects of scholarly inquiry with which to study the past. In this way, the medical fathers connect the historiographical practices of antiquity with the scholarly taxonomies of the present.

THE MEDICAL FATHERS – A EUROPEAN INVENTION?

So where *did* the notion of the medical fathers come from? My initial suspicions naturally fell on the modern pioneers of Chinese medical history, particularly Joseph Needham. In part, such suspicions were aroused by the patent anachronism of most claims about the fathers, claims that assumed the existence of something called "clinical science," "anesthesia," and "rationality" in ancient China. Indeed, such claims led me to question whether "Chinese medical history" was merely the invention of some modern scholar, ransacking the textual record for references to healers, in search of historical "data" that fit with a preconceived story inspired by European history.

That blame would fall on the modern historian is predictable enough; the influence of postcolonial studies within the China field has been rather pronounced over the last two decades. Responding to the publication of Edward Saïd's call to arms, such works take as their starting point the idea that "the ethnological thinking of the present has roots in a colonial past."[13] In the context of Chinese studies, such a paradigm has prompted scholars to trace the genealogies of modern categories and disciplines. In so doing, pervasive concepts like Confucianism have been unmasked as European inventions, the result of scholars imposing European investigative modalities onto the raw data of the Chinese past.[14]

In large part, my initial thinking about the medical fathers was guided by two studies that exemplify the genealogical approach within the China field. The first is a celebrated study, *Art in China* (1997) by Craig

Clunas, which tackles a problem that offers a rough analogy to the medical fathers. In this, Clunas makes a case against the prevailing trend of assuming the existence of something called "Chinese art," an assumption omnipresent in the opening of galleries, the writing of art history, and the organization of museums. According to Clunas, "Chinese art" was the product of scholars in nineteenth-century Europe and North America, who lumped together a diverse collection of objects produced by dissimilar parties and divergent cultural economies.[15]

The second is Lionel Jensen's *Manufacturing Confucianism* (1997), a seminal work that challenged historians to rethink the characterization of Confucius 孔子 (551–479 BC) as a philosopher.[16] According to Jensen, current understandings of this ancient figure should be understood primarily as an artifact of European modernity. Beginning in the sixteenth century, the Jesuit missionaries at court designated their hero as a pagan philosopher, on par with Plato and Aristotle, as opposed to a religious figure. Such a decision, Jensen argues, reflected the dynamics of contemporary European discourse rather than the contents of the *Analects* or the beliefs of Confucian followers. By referring to Confucius as a secular philosopher, the Jesuits effectively avoided the suggestion that the literate tradition they so admired represented a false, pagan religion. Adopted by Enlightenment philosophers, such a designation was later reintroduced into China by Western-educated modernizers during the colonial era. And it was these modernizers who awarded Confucius a prominent place in the new discipline of Chinese philosophy.[17]

Initially, Needham's medical fathers seemed to fit with the case of Chinese art or philosophy. Such a grouping gave every sign of being the result of modern historians forcing European taxonomies upon ancient textual materials. To begin with, Needham's habit of comparing Chinese figures to Hippocrates and Galen (AD 130–200), a habit he shared with other twentieth-century historians, looked like a smoking gun. Such a move offered a parallel to the Jesuit designation of Confucius as a philosopher. In addition, the stories told by twentieth-century historians bear the imprint of modernist assumptions regarding the evolution of human societies and the development of science. Take the claims about Attendant He, which I sharply criticized in an earlier article. According to Needham, this figure laid the groundwork for the advance of science from religion.[18] But this claim, I emphasized, also resembled an older, now largely discredited, narrative often told about Greek medicine in the twentieth century – to wit, that a scientific medicine required the rejection of traditional beliefs regarding the divine sources of illness. Such a resemblance, I thought, suggested that twentieth-century historians were using Chinese sources to flesh out a European theoretical skeleton – in this case, a teleological story about the development of modern science.[19]

I ultimately found the conventional explanation unsatisfactory. Such an explanation, I came to realize, was vulnerable to two recurring criticisms of works undertaken in the postcolonial vein. The first is the problem of native agency. According to critics, the singular focus on the circumstances surrounding the European construction of the Chinese past leaves the indigenous scholar out of the picture. As Thomas Trautmann puts it bluntly, such a focus leads to a "'White men in the tropics' kind of story."[20] Yet, we know that native agency was present in moments of European contact and even conquest.[21] To return to the subject of Chinese philosophy, more recent scholarship has illuminated the fact that the Jesuits could not have invented Confucius as a philosopher on their own. Such an invention, in fact, required the help of native literati, who assisted the Jesuits in their project of learning, translating, and introducing the classical canon to European audiences.[22]

Second, the postcolonial approach has been roundly criticized for overlooking the ways that non-Western systems of knowledge have shaped current scholarly practice. As Philip Wagoner sums it up, this approach assumes that there can be no significant continuities across the ruptures generated by the introduction of European epistemologies. It posits that whatever traditions of learning existed before European contact were effectively displaced by European theories. But as some historians of Indian history have forcefully pointed out, this picture of the genesis of modern disciplines has its pitfalls. By focusing exclusively on European origins, it obscures the *dual* parentage of modern scholarship – the fact that it was the conjuncture of Western *and* non-Western traditions that produced the categories, historical subjects, and theoretical resources assumed by Western scholars in the present. For example, Trautmann argues that the modern notion of the language family, a foundational idea of modern linguistics, came out of the marriage of Indian traditions of linguistic analysis to biblical ideas about genealogy.[23]

While China historians have yet to forcefully challenge narratives of rupture, there is reason to look for evidence of cross-pollination in contemporary scholarship.[24] With respect to Chinese philosophy, the Jesuits were not the first to apply an anachronistic label to Confucius. As Wiebke Denecke points out, Han dynasty bibliographers assigned Confucius to the masters category (*zi* 子) centuries after his death.[25] Such a move also had ramifications for how people read the *Analects*, having effectively lumped texts of disparate genres and provenance into a single category. More crucially, Han systems of classification were not displaced by Jesuit taxonomies; in fact, recent scholarship has highlighted the lingering influence of such classification systems on modern understandings of the past.[26] As a result, it is worth considering the extent to which Han classification systems paved the way for miscellaneous works to be relabeled as a monolithic Chinese philosophy in the early modern period. In other words, the concoction of Confucius as a philosopher was probably a collaborative effort, one that drew upon the efforts of Han bibliographers, Jesuit missionaries, and Chinese modernizers.

Indeed, if we resume our discussion of the Chinese medical fathers, there are signs that they were more than a projection of the European imagination. Granted, scholars usually trace the roots of the Chinese medical history field back to the 1920s, a period of modernization and Westernization.[27] In addition, the word now commonly used in Chinese for "medical history" (*yixue shi* 醫學史) is a modern neologism, a translation of a European term into Japanese dating to the late nineteenth century.[28] Yet as Wu Yiyi points out, before the twentieth century, "there had been a tradition in China of collecting and collating biographical data about doctors."[29]

More importantly, the medical fathers grouping was anticipated in the earliest surviving treatise on acupuncture (see Figure 2). Its early medieval author, Huangfu Mi, one of Needham's medical fathers, described the genesis of the curative arts in the following way. "In high antiquity," he wrote, "the Way of Medicine began when the Divine Husbandman (*Shennong* 神農) tasted the plants in order to learn of the hundred medicines." With this statement, Huangfu Mi recounted the deeds and discoveries of subsequent generations of healers. Following the Divine Husbandman, there was the Yellow Emperor (*Huangdi* 黃帝), who resumed the enterprise by investigating the human body with other ancient worthies; the minister of the Shang 商 dynasty (sixteenth through eleventh century BC) who committed his understanding of pharmacology to writing; and four famous court physicians who lived prior to the imperial unification of 221 BC, including the legendary Bian Que and Attendant He; last were three exemplary healers from the Han dynasty, Chunyu Yi, Hua Tuo, and Zhang Ji.[30]

Huangfu Mi's sketch resembles those of modern historians, including Needham and Lu, on several counts. To begin with, its list of exemplary healers overlaps with the aforementioned medical fathers and others to a surprising extent (though Needham, unlike his immediate predecessors,

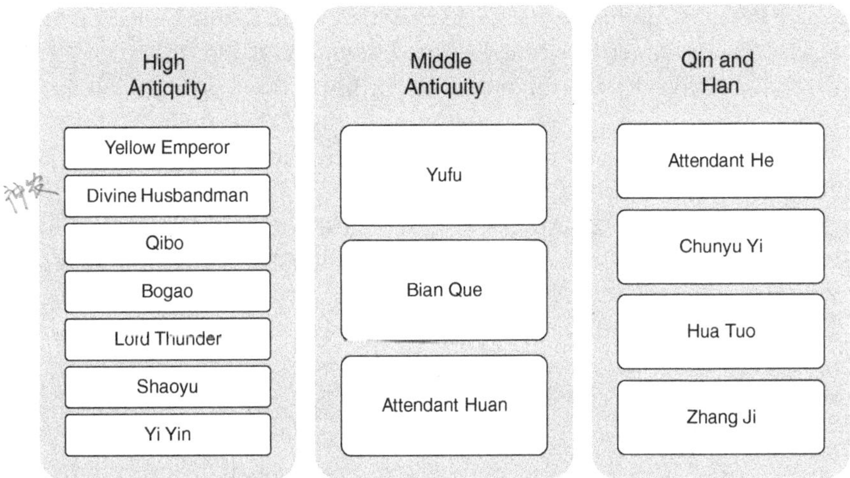

Figure 2 Huangfu Mi's list of exemplary healers. Huangfu Mi's list overlaps significantly with the narrative found in works by twentieth-century historians such as Joseph Needham.

Source: Figure drawn by author.

omitted the earliest mythical figures from his genealogy). The similarities, however, go beyond the list of figures. Like the history by Needham and Lu, Huangfu Mi chose to *illustrate* the Way of Medicine by tracing its genesis and historical evolution through exemplary figures: the cultural progenitor who discovered the curative properties of drugs, the mythical lord whose discovery of the body's mysteries enabled acupuncture, the seer who perfected the art of diagnosing incipient ills, and even a virtuoso of dubious character who practiced the arts of extending life alongside surgery. By focusing on lore about exemplary healers, Huangfu Mi's history anchored his undefined subject matter to particular moments in time and place. This history, finally, supplied human faces to what were otherwise a dizzying array of practices, texts, and techniques.

Taking the resonances between Needham and Huangfu Mi as its point of departure, the *Art of Healing in Early China* provides the first full-length study of the historiography of Chinese curative traditions. By tracing the changing boundaries of the medical archive over two millennia, this book attempts to build upon the critical spirit that animates studies in the genealogical vein, particularly those by Clunas and Jensen. It interrogates the concept of medical history – specifically, *what* has been branded medical history, and by whom? In what contexts were representations of such figures made, and what range of purposes did they serve before being combined into a single narrative? Through such methods of analysis, this book retrieves the diversity of contexts that produced stories about the medical fathers, contexts often lost or obscured by modern taxonomies.

At the same time, this book departs from the dominant focus on European modernity and its investigative modalities. Toward this end, it adopts an expanded time frame and traces the formation of the medical archive in key moments in antiquity as well as in modern times. By conducting a deep genealogy of knowledge, the *Art of Medicine* unearths the role played by ancient and medieval scholars in generating modern knowledge about the past. In this way, it invites scholars to reflect on the ways ancient and medieval forms of Chinese knowledge production are folded into the practices of modern historiography.

More concretely, the *Art of Medicine* demonstrates that the modern historiography did not emerge out of a vacuum in the 1920s. Predicated on earlier efforts to construct a medical past, this undertaking was initiated neither by Western nor by Western-educated Chinese scholars. Instead, it was an ancient philologist, the imperial bibliographer of the Han dynasty, Liu Xiang 劉向 (77–6 BC), who laid the groundwork for defining the archive of Chinese medical history. As we will see, Liu Xiang's first medical history is best thought of as a *bricolage*, a narrative cobbled together from a patchwork of repurposed textual resources. Before that time, what existed was *not* medical history but the isolated elements of one: stories about healers found in texts of dissimilar dates, authors, and aims. It was only later, in the first century BC, that such diverse materials had the status of medical history thrust upon them by Liu Xiang. Though anachronistic, Liu Xiang's taxonomy nevertheless proved to be a useful one. Providing a prototype for generations of healers and scholars to come, it was subsequently expanded upon and adapted to a range of divergent ends. Seen from this perspective, twentieth-century interpretations of medical history did *not* represent a profound break with earlier historiographical practices. On the contrary, such interpretations were merely the latest cycle of creation and destruction.

RESEARCH DESIGN

Having laid out the goals and methods of the *Art of Medicine*, I should explain how I will prove my main hypothesis: which stories about ancient healers will guide the discussion, why I have chosen them, and how I will read them.

With respect to which figures will be subject to analysis, the number of potential candidates is long. Fourteen figures are found, for example, in Huangfu Mi's barebones story alone (see Figure 2). Naturally, it is neither feasible nor desirable to give equal attention to all of the ancient figures or the stories associated with them. As a result, decisions about which figures and stories would be discussed in this book had to be made. In general, I have used two criteria for selection. First, the stories and figures must be capable of sustaining my efforts to retrieve the different contexts in which representations of ancient healers were produced. What this means, in actual practice, is that I pay scant attention to hazy mythical figures such as the Yellow Emperor. Although numerous references to this figure survive, they are too brief, or better still, too nebulous, to allow us to reconstruct the process by which an image of the medical past took shape. In addition, my discussion focuses on figures and episodes that reveal the connections between ancient histories of healing and modern historiography. For this reason, I pay attention to more proximate figures, such as Attendant He, Bian Que, Chunyu Yi, and Zhang Ji, who unlike the Yellow Emperor and the Divine Husbandman, remain staples of modern histories of medicine.

One might wonder whether there is something contradictory about my efforts to trace the archive's creation when so much of my discussion will revolve around Needham's medical fathers. In this regard, it is worth noting that my discussion departs from Needham and others primarily in terms of what goals my study hopes to achieve. By and large, previous scholars have analyzed representations of ancient healers for medical content, how medicine was practiced and what theories of the body existed, for instance. This is not an approach that will be adopted in this study. The healing arts and careers of ancient healers only figure peripherally into this study. Instead, I use the sources to explain how *representations* of ancient healers were reinterpreted as medical history. In actual practice, this means lavishing attention on the texture, form, and rhetoric of my sources while deploying the philologist's arsenal of tricks: close analyses of the language of the representations, examinations of the contexts and genres in which they appear, and investigations of figures as they move across commentarial traditions and acquire new significance and functionality.

The use of the heuristic *bricolage* to capture the ways textual matter was recycled and repurposed also bears mention. In contemporary scholarship, the term is often used loosely for any cultural product that comprises recycled material, particularly texts.[31] Charlotte Furth, for example, has characterized medical treatises of the Song 宋 dynasty (AD 960–1279) in this way, because such treatises were assembled from existing textual resources.[32] This reading does have its place in my story, for it illustrates how many early medical texts were stitched together from different materials. Yet my use of *bricolage* is broader than the sense of a mash-up, as I use the term to capture the complex conception of agency suggested by Claude Lévi-Strauss's discussion of the *bricolage* in *Savage Thought*. In this work, Lévi-Strauss pits the *bricolage* against the engineering project. Whereas the engineer first conceives of a project and then locates the resources best suited for it, the *bricoleur* works with whatever is at hand, choosing to repurpose existing materials that bear no relationship to the current project. In other words, the tools and materials employed by the *bricoleur* are *endogenous* to the current project, so their qualities cannot be explained by the goals or designs of the *bricoleur*. To understand the process by which the *bricolage* and its constitutive elements took shape, one must also consider earlier cycles of construction out of which the *bricoleur's* stock of resources arose.[33] Bearing this model of cultural production for the early Chinese case in mind, I propose to broaden our field of vision to include parties who originally had little interest in medicine: this means investigating the motives of earlier writers who furnished the stuff of which medical histories were made, as well as the contexts in which healers came to appropriate such resources.

The nettlesome term *yi* 醫, variously rendered *medicine*, *doctor*, and *physician*, merits comment. *Medicine* is an imperfect but common rendering of *yi*. Throughout this book, I will adopt this convention, with the caveat that the term should not be confused with the modern, professional variants of medicine that dominate contemporary life. The classical Chinese term was somewhat broader. From the late first century BC, authors used *yi* to cover the range of techniques related to the body, including those falling largely outside the boundaries of modern Western medicine: exorcisms, invocations, fasting and dietetics, meditation, sexual abstinence and manipulations, breathing exercises, and gymnastics. What is more, such techniques did not merely pertain to healing, for they also purportedly promoted vitality and longevity.[34]

In addition, I will resist the common translation of *yi* as *doctor* and *physician*. In some cases, such a translation makes sense. Some of the men and women referred to as *yi* were in fact celebrity healers with extensive training in the curative arts, and they earned a living and reputation through healing. But care must be taken not to conflate the classical term with the modern, narrow sense of an M.D., a member of a prestigious and well-remunerated profession.[35] Healers in early and medieval

China did *not* band together as a collective social group, let alone as a profession: an autonomous, self-regulating organization that fixed standards, set fees, or controlled its membership.[36] To quote Nathan Sivin, "Physicians of the small literate office-holding class never saw themselves as part of a larger group that included priestly ritual healers, sellers of *materia medica*, therapists of various kinds who might or might not be able to read and write, folk wonder-workers, and so on."[37]

That *yi* should not be confused with career healers bears emphasis here. The potential for confusion reflects the fact that the classical Chinese graph is the same one used in the modern term *yisheng* 醫生 (*physician, doctor*). In addition, the language of our sources is sometimes misleading. Some passages in classical texts use the term in an indefinite sense even when referring to specific groups of healers. An oft-quoted remark from a canonical work on ritual, compiled in the first century BC, offers one such example. It admonishes gentlemen to "avoid becoming familiar" with healers (*yi*), invocators, craftsmen, and other lowlifes.[38] Though such remarks are easily interpreted as evidence of general attitudes toward *yi*, the larger context must be borne in mind, for their author intended them to refer more specifically to certain kinds of healers: those of marginal status, such as the men and women who peddled drugs in the marketplaces or tended to abscesses.

Instead, the classical Chinese term *yi* is best understood as a blanket label for anyone who practiced or wrote about the diverse arts related to the upkeep of the body.[39] This included the illiterate, humble men who made their living by attending to the physical woes of others. But it applied also to the men and women who held medical posts inside the Han bureaucracy: the attendants at court who tended to the wounds of rulers; the county officers who applied moxa and acupuncture to the sick;[40] members of the frontier army who distributed, prepared, and kept track of the supply of medicine in the provinces and frontiers;[41] and the women who oversaw the nursing of imperial children.[42] Given its broad and relatively indefinite scope, *yi* invites comparisons with the contemporary English word *musician*, a term so general as to encompass street performers, cabaret singers, esteemed maestros, recording artists, and members of high school orchestra bands. For these reasons, my translation of *yi* will vary depending on context. In cases in which the person in question looked after the well-being of the body, particularly in the absence of illness, I will opt for the more open-ended translation of *yi* as *attendant*. In other cases, in which the person treated the ills of the body, I render the term as *healer* – regardless of the practitioner's status or level of training.

OVERVIEW

Each of the six chapters traces different aspects of the ancient medical archive. The first half of this book looks at representations of exemplary healers before the emergence of "medical history." It attempts to retrieve the historical and rhetorical contexts that produced representations of these figures. In contrast, the second half examines the formation of medical histories in early and medieval China through the exemplary healer list. It shows that the present image of the early medical fathers was produced in response to different events before the twentieth century: the reorganization of the imperial collections in 26 BC, the rise of literati healers beginning in the Song dynasty, the publication of important medical classics in the 1060s, and the emergence of textual controversies regarding a canonical work of medicine.

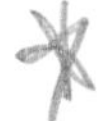

The first chapter, "Attendant He: Innovator or Persona?," investigates one personality, the Qin 秦 healer, Attendant He 和. Historians have treated the episode featuring Attendant He in one chronicle, the *Tradition of Zuo* (*Zuozhuan* 左傳), as a source for medical practice in antiquity. This chapter proposes that this interpretation is at variance with the figure's original function in the text. By analyzing the narrative structure of the *Tradition of Zuo*, it argues that Attendant He served as a literary device in the original narrative. The beliefs attributed to him in that account further conformed to an archetypal representation found in various chronicles, the noble expert of the numinous realm. Consequently, one should think of the figure as the work of chroniclers, who were concerned primarily with political matters, and for whom healing represented an afterthought.

Chapter 2 or "Bian Que as a Seer" also examines a celebrated episode still used by historians to explain the theories of ancient healers. Bian Que, cast as the protagonist of this particular annal, is often used to illuminate the emphasis on preventive care within the Chinese medical tradition. By tracing the earliest surviving version of the episode to a political treatise, this chapter shows that Bian Que is best thought of as the creation of the court persuaders in the Warring States period (453–221 BC). Such persuaders reworked the figure to make a rhetorical point (about the importance of rooting out political ills) rather than to provide a model of diagnosis. It was only much later that this story was reinterpreted in a biographical light.

The first two chapters reveal how modern histories of medicine drew upon sources that bore only a tangential relationship to the curative arts and ancient healers. Chapter 3, "Chunyu Yi: Can the Healer Speak?," revisits evidence that suggests that practitioners of the curative arts also contributed to the modern historian's archive. It does so by focusing on the biography of the Granary Master (comp. ca. 90 BC), which includes twenty-five records of medical consultation attributed to a historical figure, Chunyu Yi. Here, the chapter argues that the records were in part the work of someone who practiced the arts of healing. But this does not imply that such records were either composed by career healers or for the purpose of constructing a medical history. Instead, the form and style worked toward the goal of translating medical knowledge into a bureaucratic idiom. Such translations, moreover, often occurred when healers recorded their efforts to treat illness in an administrative context. The move to interpret such records as medical documents – or the impulse to mine them for their therapeutic or genealogical value – represents a later development.

Whereas the first three chapters focus on the elements constitutive of the exemplary healer list, the fourth chapter turns to the matter of when authors began to weave materials found in disparate textual traditions into a coherent origins story. It argues that the first origins story derived from the imperial bibliographer Liu Xiang. Though elements of Liu Xiang's narrative were anticipated several centuries before his time, the practice of bringing all of these voices together into a single list of exemplary healers emerged surprisingly late: in the first century BC and as a result of Liu Xiang's efforts to reorganize the imperial collections. Despite the fact that Liu Xiang was neither a healer nor an acknowledged medical ancestor, his narrative equipped later medieval healers with a template for writing medical histories. Understood from this perspective, the initial creation of an exemplary healer list owed much to the new ways of engaging the past that accompanied the reorganization of the imperial collections.

The fifth chapter, "Zhang Ji: The Kaleidoscopic Father," moves our story beyond the Han. It questions the extent to which the lore attached to the medical fathers remained fixed in medieval times. To answer this question, my discussion turns to the legendary healer Zhang Ji, an important figure in the medical traditions of medieval and late imperial times. In modern accounts, Zhang Ji is often presented as a tragic figure, who took up the study of medicine in response to a well-documented epidemic that wiped out his family. As shown through a survey of medieval sources, this personality developed over time, emerging in view only in the eleventh century. The changes in Zhang Ji's image, furthermore, can be traced back to a pivotal event, the emergence of elite healers during the Song dynasty, who practiced medicine as a trade and for whom the past was key for defining their legitimacy. Such healers made opportunistic use of a story found in a preface published by the Song Imperial Bureau of Editing Texts in 1065, a preface that inadvertently took shape during the process of transmission. Seizing upon the story, such healers remade Zhang Ji in the image of Confucius, thereby bolstering claims that the curative arts represented a counterpart to the classics and thus a pursuit befitting of gentlemen. In this way, the case of Zhang Ji reveals how the shape of the medical archive owed as much to medieval healers as to ancient bibliographers.

The final chapter, "Huangfu Mi: From Innovator to Transmitter," investigates the implications of the archive's medieval reorderings for modern historians. The previous chapter showed that the medical fathers acquired new meanings and functions over time. This, however, leaves a question: to what extent did subsequent reorderings result in the loss of earlier meanings? This chapter investigates shifting representations of Huangfu Mi, who is largely presented today as the editor of ancient works, rather than a medical innovator or master healer in his own right. Yet Huangfu Mi's image was as unstable as Zhang Ji's. In the first half of the medieval period, early authors depicted Huangfu Mi as a man, chronically ill, and associated with a controversial drug. Later, in the Song dynasty, Huangfu Mi ended up acquiring a reputation as an erudite editor who transmitted ancient works of dubious provenance. Although modern presentations of Huangfu Mi have followed portrayals influenced by his Song transmigration, vestiges of his earlier persona persist. Such a persona, in fact, was rediscovered in the twentieth century and marshaled by the opponents of opium.

The Epilogue, "Ancient Histories in the Modern Age," takes us to more recent accounts of medical history. The twentieth century is often seen as a watershed moment in Chinese medical history, but to what extent do modern retellings reproduce the logic of earlier historiographical practices? By focusing on several of the medical fathers who figure prominently in twentieth-century retellings, the epilogue argues that while they emphasize different themes, twentieth-century presentations also exhibit some striking continuities with earlier accounts. Indeed, these modern histories might also be thought of as *bricolage*. The men who wrote them did not fashion new narratives from scratch. Together with their classically literate collaborators, they instead articulated new histories of Chinese medicine not only by recycling bits and pieces of premodern accounts, but also by channeling the early medical fathers.

Taken together, the six chapters and epilogue reveal that the introduction of modern European ideologies and frameworks to China did not simply replace the knowledge systems of earlier eras. Acknowledged or not, the work of ancient philologists and medieval editors lives on in the present, embedded in current visions of medical history.

PART I

BEFORE MEDICAL HISTORY

1

ATTENDANT HE: INNOVATOR OR PERSONA?

As attendant he did not belong to a hazy antiquity, it is no accident that Needham began his story about Chinese medicine with the sixth-century figure.[1] Unlike the other exemplary healers found in Huangfu Mi's preface, whose names signaled their mythical quality – the Divine Husbandman, the Yellow Emperor, and Lord Thunder (*Leigong* 雷公) – Attendant He gave every appearance of being historical. Judging from ancient chronicles, he served as some kind of medical attendant in the western state of Qin centuries before the unification of China in 221 BC. One can furthermore pinpoint his activities in time, as he traveled in 541 BC to the state of Jin 晉 to attend to the sick Lord Ping 平. A detailed record of Attendant He's diagnosis of that lord, moreover, survives in the *Tradition of Zuo*, a historical chronicle by an unknown author.

Not surprisingly, modern scholars assume that Attendant He was a *historical* personage, and they recount his contributions to medical theory as if the ancient man were Herophilus (335–ca. 280 BC) or William Harvey (1578–1657). A recent history by Zhu Jianping 朱建平 serves as a case in point. Before Attendant He, Zhu writes, "illness was seen as heavenly sanction or a scourge sent down by the spirits"; after Attendant He, illness "could be analyzed solely in terms of material causes." This rejection of superstition, Zhu further adds, provided "the conceptual breakthrough for the foundations of the theory of pathogenesis found in the *Yellow Emperor's Inner Classic*."[2]

Similar conjectures about Attendant He's historicity surface in important Japanese- and English-language works on Chinese medicine, where scholars treat the healer as a representative of new theories that connected human health and sickness to cosmic patterns.[3] Japanese scholar, Yamada Keiji, for instance, assumes that the description of Attendant He in the *Tradition of Zuo* is historical and characterizes the episode as the first evidence of medicine as a system of knowledge.[4] Similarly, in his celebrated study, the *Expressiveness of the Body*, Kuriyama Shigehisa also regards Attendant He as a historical figure. The healer, Kuriyama asserts, "ignored demonic attacks, but instead blamed six causes: the *yin*, the *yang*, wind, rain, darkness, and brightness."[5]

Yet should one treat the episode in the *Tradition of Zuo* as China's first medical case history? Does it actually reveal what Attendant He or, for that matter, what any ancient healer believed? Admittedly, the chronicle relates events in the regional courts of the Spring and Autumn (ca. 771–453 BC), the time of Attendant He's heyday. Yet most scholars now agree that the text postdated the Spring and Autumn by centuries. In the mid-fourth century BC, a chronicler reworked earlier materials and pieces of legend to express his understanding of the moral patterns of the past. In the process, he adapted and added fictionalized speeches, episodes, and entire personalities.[6] The chronicler also happened to be a master of narrative. Like a novelist or bard, he availed himself of an arsenal of rhetorical devices to drive home his larger message: rhymed speeches, prolepsis, dream narration, fictional episodes, and fantastic elements such as visits by ghosts and demons.[7] Given all of these features, it seems unwise to assume that the historical figure of Attendant He, if he existed, was just as he appeared in the *Tradition of Zuo*.

This chapter revisits the famous episode preserved in the *Tradition of Zuo*. It challenges a basic assumption underlying most modern interpretations of Attendant He's significance: namely, that the episode in the *Tradition of Zuo* provides a mirror of medical thinking and practice in ancient China. As shall be shown in the following text, one should not think of the figure as a historical person as much as a persona: a fictional character that the anonymous chronicler created for purposes of narrative intensification. The chronicler, furthermore, I will argue, recounted the episode to relate a political parable rather than to record a momentous event in Chinese medical history.

To show this, I begin by introducing the episode in the *Tradition of Zuo*: explaining its historical context, main characters, and key themes before providing a synopsis. I then revisit the episode, attempting to establish the kind of character Attendant He represented in the narrative. Through these methods, I argue that contrary to conventional wisdom, the chronicler represented the healer as both an authority on the body and an expert on the numinous realm. With such a reevaluation, I situate the healer's prognosis within the larger story about Lord Ping's illness. By analyzing the narrative structure, I demonstrate that the chronicler presented Attendant He as the alter ego of another figure in the episode, a statesman renowned for his knowledge of spiritual matters. The views that the chronicler attributed to the figure moreover fit with a common archetype in Warring States histories, that being the noble master of the numinous realm. For this reason, I conclude that the chronicler fashioned the image of the healer by recycling existing tropes and archetypes to make a point about politics, as opposed to medicine.

SETTING THE STAGE

Before going too much further, it would be helpful to place the episode examined in the following discussion in its historical context, as well as to introduce its main themes and characters. The episode in the *Tradition of Zuo* purportedly took place around 541 BC, an era that scholars refer to as the Spring and Autumn (ca. 771–453 BC). The period acquired its name from a famous annals traditionally attributed to Confucius, which narrates political events from the perspective of the Master's home state of Lu 魯. At the start of the Spring and Autumn period, there were literally hundreds of states in China proper. Centuries of warfare, however, reduced the number of states to only a handful of superpowers. In the sixth century BC, the state of Jin was one of a number of superpowers, along with Qi 齊 in the East, Qin 秦 in the West, and Chu 楚 in the South, that vied for hegemonic status. (For a map of the period, see Figure 3.)

The main subject and *dramatis personae* of the episode also bear mention. Told from the perspective of multiple figures at court, the chronicler's narrative revolved around the sickness of Lord Ping. In it, the chronicler explored both the specific and general roots of the illness, whether the sickness was the result of meddling angry spirits, or if the unhealthy lifestyle of the lord contributed to his malaise. In addition, the chronicler teased out the political implications of the lord's sickness – what, for instance, the lord's sickness revealed about the quality of ministers, the future of the ruling house, and the governance of the state. Besides Lord Ping, three figures played a central role in the episode: Lord Ping's chief minister Zhao Wu 趙武 (d. 541 BC); Zichan 子產 (d. 522), a famous nobleman and an emissary from the smaller state of Zheng 鄭 to Jin's south; and Attendant He, the medical attendant from Qin.

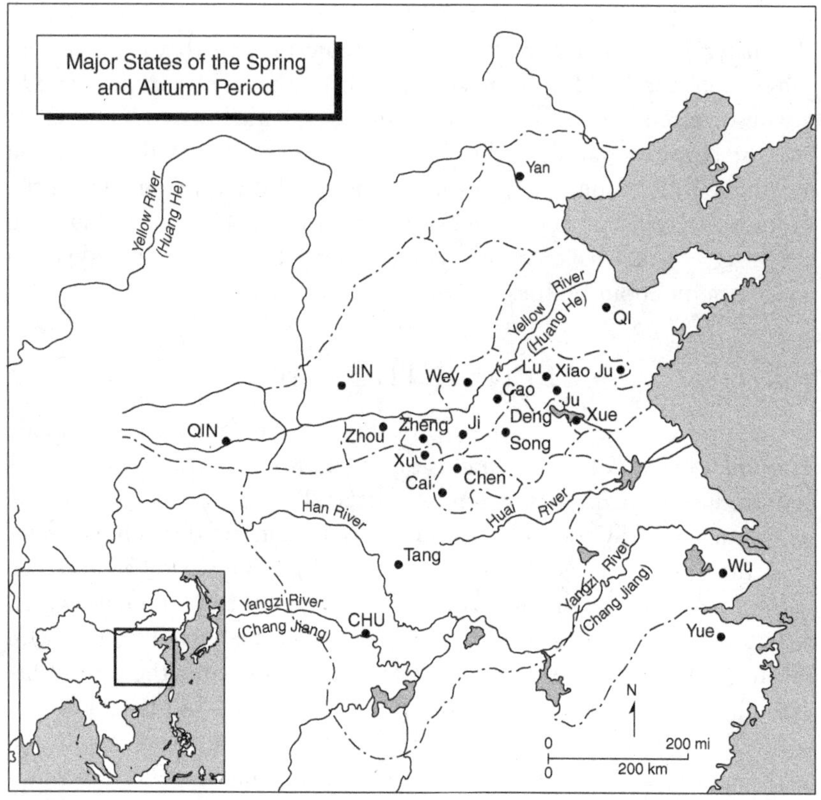

Figure 3 Major states during the Spring and Autumn period, ca. 771–453 BC.

Source: The Cambridge History of Ancient China: From the Origins of Civilization to 221 BC, edited by Michael Loewe and Edward L. Shaughnessy, 548 (1999). Reproduced with permission from Cambridge University Press.

The chronicler narrated the episode, represented in Figures 4 and 5, through two events: first, Zichan's mission to the Jin court and his conversations about Lord Ping's illness; and second, Attendant He's visit to Jin and his remarks about the roots of the lord's sickness.

Upon closer inspection, one can see that the narrative about Zichan's visit is in fact tripartite. The first part opens with the arrival of Zichan in Jin, where a divination had just been performed to determine the etiology of Lord Ping's illness. The diviners at the Jin court reported that two spirits were behind the sickness. Because no one in the Jin court was familiar with the spirits, Zichan was asked about them. Much to the surprise of his audience, Zichan flatly denied that the spirits were

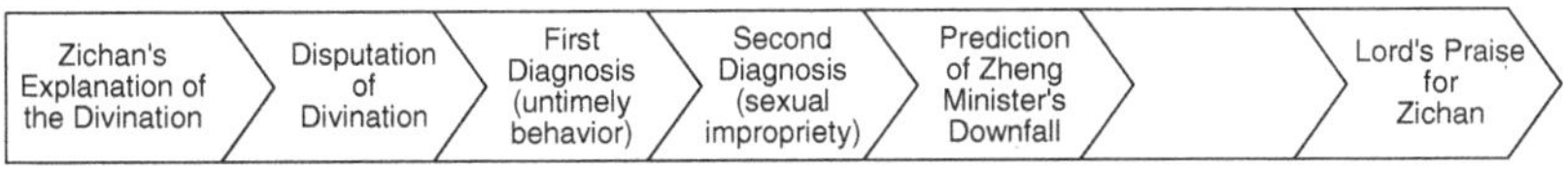

Figure 4 The Sickness of Lord Ping at a Glance (Zichan), as recorded in the *Tradition of Zuo* (4th cent. BC). The diagram schematically represents Zichan's mission to Jin.

Source: Image drawn by author.

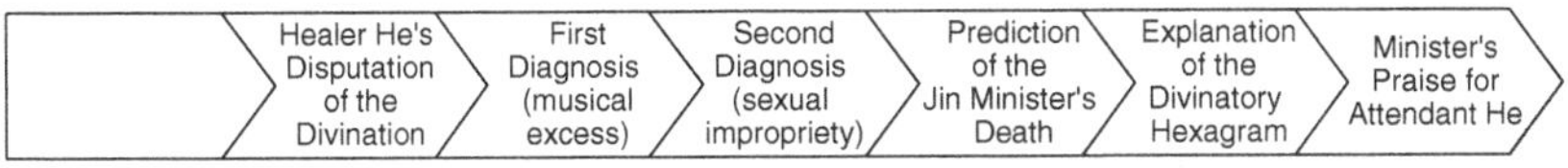

Figure 5 The Sickness of Lord Ping at a Glance (Attendant He), as recorded in the *Tradition of Zuo* (4th cent. BC). The diagram analyzes the visit of Attendant He.

Source: Image drawn by author.

involved. The pair, Zichan explained, were nature spirits and did not have dominion over the lord's body. "What do the gods of the hills and rivers, or of the stars and planets," he asked, "have to do with the health of the prince?" The real source of the lord's illness, Zichan explained, came down to two factors: first, the lord's disorderly lifestyle, which was at odds with the proper time for activities, and second, his flagrant violation of taboos against marrying women of the same surname.[8]

In the second part of Zichan's visit, the chronicler moved away from Zichan to a conversation between a Jin noble and another member of the Zheng delegation. This Jin nobleman inquired about the chief minister of Zichan's home state of Zheng, to which the delegate replied that the days of the Zheng minister in question were numbered. In the third and shortest part, the chronicler returned to Lord Ping of Jin, who listened to the prognosis before bestowing words of praise and tokens of appreciation upon Zichan.[9]

The second event can also be divided into roughly three parts. The first and longest opens with Attendant He's consultation with his noble patient, Lord Ping, where the healer rejected the possibility that either ghosts or bad food had caused the illness. "There is nothing that can be done," he told the lord, "For this is what is referred to as a case of 'being close to women,' a sickness generated in the same way as *gu* 蠱."[10] After announcing his prognosis, Attendant He then issued a mysterious prophecy about the imminent death of a minister in the Jin court (I say mysterious because the healer did not identify the doomed minister by name). The prophecy, however, was ignored by the lord, who was more worried about the prospect of having to abandon his riotous lifestyle.

Instead, Lord Ping got back to what really mattered. "Is it true," he asked Attendant He, "that women are not to be approached?" The question gave the healer an opening to lecture the rakish lord on the roots of illness: excessive indulgence in music and unregulated sexual activity. According to Attendant He, Lord Ping's sexual excess had caused an imbalance in the body, which had made the lord sick.

In the second part, the chronicler turned his attention away from the consultation between the patient and healer to a conversation between the latter and Minister Zhao Wu. The latter had learned from someone that Attendant He had issued a prophecy regarding the imminent death of an unnamed minister. Evidently intrigued, or perhaps worried, Minister Zhao demanded that the healer identify the minister in question, only to hear that it was he. As the conversation had taken an awkward turn, Minister Zhao changed the subject and asked instead about the illness called *gu*, mentioned by Attendant He in his preceding remarks. In response, Attendant He explained the illness through passages drawn from the divinatory classic, the *Book of Zhou Changes* (*Zhouyi* 周易 or *Yi-ching*). In the third and briefest part, the chronicler closed with Minister Zhao's words of praise for Attendant He, who was extolled as a "fine healer" and rewarded for his visit to Jin.[11]

WHO WAS HE?

With such an introduction, we now return to the primary problem at hand: investigating whether or not the episode in the *Tradition of Zuo* was actually a literal account of medical happenings. For this, one must first acquire a deeper understanding of the medical figure in the *Tradition of Zuo*. Was Attendant He, as many historians argue, a naturalist? And by naturalist, they mean that the healer had excluded supernatural forces like gods and spirits from his accounts of sickness, instead explaining illness in terms of the metaphysical frameworks concerned with expressions of *qi*, and the balance between *yin* and *yang*. Though present in virtually all modern discussions, the received view about Attendant He, I think, misses the mark. Although he associated Attendant He with *qi*-centered theories of illness, the chronicler also presented the man as an expert of the spirit realm – a point that will be crucial for my larger argument about the healer functioning as a literary device in the text.

At first blush, the evidence would seem to favor the received view. Nowhere in his prognosis did Attendant He mention the spirits, and so it would seem that the chronicler rendered him a proponent of naturalistic theories of illness. This would seem obvious enough from the text of the healer's celebrated prognosis.

> 天有六氣，降生五味，發為五色，徵為五聲。淫生六疾。六氣曰陰、陽、風、雨、晦、明也，分為四時，序為五節，過則為菑：陰淫寒疾，陽淫熱疾，風淫末疾，雨淫腹疾，晦淫惑疾，明淫心疾。女、陽物而晦時，淫則生內熱惑蠱之疾。今君不節、不時，能無及此乎?」
>
> In Heaven there are six kinds of *qi*, which come down and produce the five flavors, emitted as the five hues, and result in the five tones. If there is excess, the six illnesses will be produced. The six *qi* are referred to as the *yin*, *yang*, wind, rain, dark, and light, each of which are separated into four periods and arranged into five pitches. When there is excess in one of these, there will be calamity. When the *yin* is excessive, there will be a cold illness, when the *yang* is excessive, there will be a heat illness; when wind is excessive, there will be an illness in the extremities; when rain is excessive, there will be an illness of the abdomen; when darkness is excessive, there will be avolition, and when light is excessive, there will be an illness in the heart. Women draw out the *yang* [i.e., the bright or hard] in things during the hours of darkness (?).[12] When there is excess in this, an internal heat, avolition, and *gu* will be produced. In the present case, I knew that his lordship had been immoderate and untimely in his sexual relations; thus how could this calamity not have befallen him?[13]

The passage presents several points of interest. To begin with, the chronicler not only excluded references to gods and spirits from Attendant He's prognosis, but he instead emphasized the cosmological underpinnings of human illness: the excesses of *yin* and *yang*, as well as the uneven proportions of dark and light or moisture and heat, all of which cause the body to lose its natural equilibrium. The very generality of the prognosis – notice, for example, that the healer brought up symptoms that the patient did not experience – suggests that Attendant He saw the theory of the six *qi* as a framework for understanding not only the illness of Lord Ping, but also human sickness in general.

Perhaps more importantly, Attendant He denied in the episode that the lord's illness resulted from the malevolent involvement of spirits.[14] Such a denial is surprising in light of other sources from the fourth century BC. If divinatory records recovered by archaeologists are any indication, illness was seen by the ruling elite as the result of supernatural displeasure: Heaven "sending down" its punishments, an ancestor or spirit miffed about having received less than his or her due of offerings, a demon seeking vengeance upon a murderer or his descendants, and the war dead incensed by a lack of sacrifices.[15] The case of one nobleman, who died a few decades after the compilation of the *Tradition of Zuo*, leaves clues as to the strength of such beliefs among the ruling elite. His ailments occasioned the coordinated efforts of twelve diviners, who sacrificed no less than thirty-six pigs, six dogs, twenty-three sheep, nine oxen, and a horse.[16] Given such a background, the healer's denial that spirits and ghosts caused the lord's illness seems all the more like an expression of defiance, a protest lodged against the dominant views of the age.

The attention that the healer purportedly gave to symptoms would also seem incompatible with conceptions of illness as divine punishment. The fact that Attendant He worked backward from symptoms to source suggests that he saw a one-to-one relationship between a symptom and the agent of illness – a stance at odds with older views that emphasized the capriciousness of spirits. While they ascribed a rationality to illness – the gods and spirits usually had a reason for sending down the scourge of sickness – older views did not posit a necessary connection between specific symptoms and agents. As divination records hinted, the expression of spiritual displeasure varied widely; the same illness could have any number of potential sources. When investigating the shortness of breath and loss of appetite suffered by the aforementioned nobleman, diviners considered a long list of candidates: royal ancestors, various nature spirits, and those who died in war.[17] Given the lack of correspondence between symptom and agent, diviners understandably paid little attention to the former, instead scrutinizing the patterns found in the turtle shells and milfoil stalks for clues about the sources of illness.

Moreover, other elements in the episode militate against the view that Attendant He opposed spiritual explanations of illness. Although he did not assign any role to the spirits in his diagnosis of Lord Ping, the healer failed to issue a categorical denial. Upon closer examination, this healer not only ruled out spirits, but also the effects of bad food. "This is not the work of ghosts," he declared, "nor the result of what was eaten" (*fei gui fei shi* 非鬼非食).[18] The scope of these oft-quoted remarks deserves explication. Did the chronicler intend them as general statements, namely, that ghosts *never* make people ill? Or was the chronicler just referring to the *particular* case of Lord Ping? Although the language of the passage is vague, the second interpretation is probably the more coherent of the two. If one reads the remarks as a blanket statement, then that would mean that Attendant He had excluded food as the source of illness *in all cases*. But that is absurd.

Worse still, the prognosis regarding Minister Zhao linked Attendant He to older views that attributed illness to spiritual displeasure. Admittedly, Attendant He did not say in so many words that the spirits could punish men or women by making them sick. But in the midst of delivering his diagnosis of Lord Ping, he abruptly changed the subject and issued the following statement: "A good minister will die, for Heaven's will does not protect him" (*tianming buyou* 天命不祐).[19] To readers unfamiliar with the literary conventions of the genre, the utterance is puzzling because it seems out of place. To start with, it sounds as if the healer issued not only a prognosis for the sick lord, but also a prophecy about another person, an unnamed minister, who would be revealed as none other than Minister Zhao. In this passage, the chronicler did not use *tianming* 天命 to refer to the more familiar sense of a dynastic mandate. Instead, the chronicler was pointing to the will of an anthropomorphic Heaven, who saw fit to visit early deaths on immoral men.[20] When pressed for details by Minister Zhao, Attendant He explained that Heaven would punish the minister with death:

> 和聞之, 國之大臣, 榮其寵祿, 任其 寵 〔大〕節。有菑禍興, 而無改焉, 必受其咎。今君至於淫以生疾, 將不能圖恤社稷, 禍孰大焉?主不能禦, 吾是以云也。」

> I, He, have also heard it said that if honored by favors and emoluments and having assumed responsibility for the gravest of state matters, the great minister makes no change to affairs when a disaster arises, he too will suffer the consequences of the spiritual fault. At present the lord has been licentious to the point that he became ill and is unable to plan for the care of the altars of earth and grain [i.e., the state]. What disaster is more serious than this? You, sir, have been unable to intervene in this matter, and so I was speaking of you.[21]

Given the importance of this passage, it is worth lingering over the chronicler's choice of words. Here, he used the term *jiu* 咎, which I have translated as "spiritual fault." In ancient texts, the term referred generally to blameworthy conduct. But ancient writers often used *jiu* to describe offenses that merited divine retribution; hence the common rendering of "curse." In fact, in ancient records of divination, scribes paired *jiu* with *sui* 祟, the sickness, misfortune, or even death meted out by baleful spirits.[22] The use of *jiu* in this way moreover makes sense given the larger context of the passage; Attendant He said that Minister Zhao would be punished for allowing the young lord to pursue the life of a rake. In other words, Heaven would execute the minister for being remiss.

Further complicating matters is Attendant He's avowed interest in divination, an interest that runs against the received view of him as a naturalist. When conversing about the prophecy, the healer was asked by the minister to expand on the meaning of the term *gu*, a term that the healer used in his prognosis of Lord Ping. Here, Attendant He reportedly explained the term by its graph. "If we look at it, we see that 'vessel' and 'worms' make *gu*." The healer then tied his interpretation of the graph to its entry in a classic of divination. "In the *Book of Zhou Changes*," he noted, "a woman deluding a man or the wind toppling a mountain is *gu*."[23] ䷑

An analysis of the healer's remarks thus reveals a figure more complex than he would initially appear. At first glance, Attendant He did seem to eschew spiritual explanations of illness, because *qi* served as the focus of the prognosis. Yet one should be wary of treating this healer as an opponent of older conceptions of illness. Had this been the case, he would not have spoken of Heavenly punishment, because such an utterance implied the power of the spirits to deliver lesser punishments like sickness. Making matters worse, the received view of Attendant He as the enemy of superstition also falters upon closer examination, for Attendant He not only issued prophecies but also presented himself as an expert on divination.

HISTORICAL PERSON OR LITERARY DEVICE?

Our foregoing discussion leaves us to question if the chronicler's presentation of Attendant He should be taken at face value. The question arises because the *Tradition of Zuo* is famous for being a "doctored" text. As noted previously, the chronicler recounted events selectively, and he crafted speeches and entire episodes to illustrate his historical and moral vision. In this regard, the episode about Lord Ping's illness was no exception. As Jin Shiqi 金仕起 points out in a brilliant article, the chronicler did not intend to expound on the finer points of medical theory but rather to explain the underlying causes behind the fall of Jin in the fifth century BC. Indeed, Jin Shiqi argues that there is little about the account that is specifically medical. He notes that Attendant He's conceptual vocabulary was indistinguishable from that of Zichan or other noble figures in the *Tradition of Zuo*.[24] Given all this, it behooves us to ask what purpose Attendant He served within the text. Through an analysis of the narrative's formal structure, I demonstrate that the chronicler created the medical figure after the image of Zichan, an important minister *and* renowned expert on spiritual matters.

The structure of the narrative about Lord Ping's illness provides the best evidence that one should regard Attendant He and Zichan as textual doubles or twins. As the bird's-eye view of the narrative found in Figures 4 and 5 shows, the two figures occupy similar positions within the symmetrical halves of the episode. To be sure, the chronicler sprinkled elements of variation to minimize the monotony of repetition. Whereas Zichan's explanation of the divination appeared early in the narrative, Attendant He deferred his discussion of the divinatory classic until the end of his speech. Discrepancies aside, the chronicler created the two halves of the narrative in parallel. Both opened with the main figure disputing the message of the diviners and providing alternative explanations of the lord's sickness. Zichan blamed the illness on the lord's use of time and concubines who shared the lord's surname, while Attendant He attributed the sickness to the lord's overindulgence in loud musical performances and sexual excess.[25] At this point, the chronicler introduced a turn or what poets call a *svolta*, which shifted the discussion away from the subject of the lord's health to the chief ministers in the states of Zheng and Jin. In each half, the chronicler closed with words of praise; Lord Ping described Zichan as a "gentleman of broad learning" and gave him a rich gift, and Minister Zhao extolled Attendant He as a "fine healer" and ordered the healer escorted back to Qin with ceremony.

Aside from such structural parallels, the doubling of Zichan and Attendant He can be seen at the level of thematic content and style. All this is unsurprising considering that Attendant He's speech closely resembled that of Zichan. Both figures rejected the conventional interpretation of the divination, and they stressed the importance of restraint in sexual matters. In addition, Zichan's emphasis on timing resonated with Attendant He's injunctions for men to know when to stop a musical performance. The use of counterfactual reasoning presents an additional similarity. Zichan ruled out the gods by exploring likely expressions of divine displeasure and clarifying the lack of connection between the spirits and the lord's sickness. As he put it, if the gods of the mountains and rivers were angry, they would bring "disasters of floods, droughts, and pestilence." And if it were the gods of the sun, moon, stars, and planets, one would expect to see "untimely snow, frost, wind, and rain." Attendant He similarly arrived at his prognosis by entertaining other scenarios before settling on a description that provided the best match: "When the *yin* is excessive, there will be a cold illness, and when the *yang* is excessive, there will be a heat illness; when wind is excessive, there will be an illness in the extremities; when rain is excessive, there will be an illness of the abdomen. . . ."

There is a final reason to regard Attendant He as the textual double of Zichan: the chronicler also used other healers as rhetorical devices.[26] The famous encounter between Huan 緩 (ca. 581 BC) and an earlier ruler of Jin provides one such example. The chronicler opened with an episode in which Lord Ping's predecessor dreamt about a vengeful ghost, who declared that the lord would be punished for having murdered the ghost's descendants. Concerned, the lord first consulted a wizard, who confirmed the correctness of the dream and added that the lord would not live to eat the new grain. So when the lord fell ill, Huan was summoned from the Qin state. Before Huan arrived, however, the lord had a second dream, in which the illness took the form of two lads residing inside of his body and discussing the imminent arrival of the healer. One said, "Huan is a fine attendant, and I fear that he will harm us and so how can we escape?" In response, the other proposed to evade the healer by moving to the area between the heart and diaphragm. "If we do this," the second lad replied, "What can he do to us?" And indeed, when he finally arrived, Huan declared the illness to be incurable. "The illness," he told the lord, "resides in the space between the heart and diaphragm," so the healer's arsenal of remedies was of no use. Hearing this, the lord praised Huan as a "fine attendant" and sent him back to his home state with pomp and ceremony. At first, the lord's condition did not worsen, leading him to believe that he had outwitted fate. Confident, the lord then recalled the wizard, showing him the new grain before killing him. But just as the lord tasted the new grain, he collapsed, dying shortly thereafter.[27] Here, the parallels between Huan's visit and the encounter with the unfortunate wizard suggest a doubling effect. As Li Wai-yee notes, the two episodes are symmetrical.[28] Structurally, both healer and wizard stood in the same relation to the lord; both conversed with him after his dream and confirmed its message. The wizard described a future that corresponded to the first dream about ghostly retribution, and the healer's prediction matched the conversation overheard in the second. Through such doubling, the chronicler introduced an element of narrative intensification, as the repetition reinforced the inevitability of the lord's end.[29]

Thus far, I have demonstrated that Attendant He and Zichan represent textual doubles, but did this mean that the healer was actually the counterpart to an expert on the spirits? The issue merits consideration, because some scholars have read this episode differently. Pointing to Zichan's invocation of *qi*, one historian argues that Zichan challenged older beliefs regarding the divine or demonic origins of illness.[30] Similarly, Aihe Wang characterizes the episode as evincing a break with Bronze Age cosmology. After this putative break, Wang proposes, the early Chinese elite ceased to regard the sicknesses of princes as signs of ancestral displeasure as much as the "expression of a cosmic pattern that regulated both natural and social orders."[31]

In fairness, Zichan (like Attendant He) did *not* deny that spirits could have produced Lord Ping's illness. Yet here Zichan instead stressed the role played by bad habits and improper sexual relations: the lord ignored the importance of adhering to rules about when to perform certain activities, instead living his life in a haphazard fashion. As Zichan explained it to his interlocutor, everything had its proper time: "The morning is when one listens to the business of governance, daytime is for visits, the dusk is for deciding upon commands, and the evening for resting the body." Such rules were hardly arbitrary, he added, for they were intended to safeguard the health of the body. By adhering to them, Zichan claimed, "one is able to temper the *qi*, thereby preventing blockages and accumulations that weaken the body, dull the heart, and bring chaos to the hundred affairs." Worse still, the lord ignored prohibitions against sexual relations with women of the same surname, prohibitions that prevented barren unions and illnesses resulting from sexual contact with relatives. "Once the initial attraction has worn off," Zichan warned, "the two people of the same surname will produce illnesses in each other."[32]

Questions aside, other evidence suggests that the chronicler presented Attendant He's textual double, Zichan, as a noble expert on the numinous realm.[33] As a point of fact, the members of the Jin court had not asked Zichan to weigh in on the sources of the illness, but rather to interpret the results of a divination. Unlike the Confucius portrayed in the *Analects*, who was famously reticent about matters involving the spirits,[34] Zichan accepted the challenge readily. He recounted the identities of the spirits – their origins, the background behind their respective domains, the states under their control, and so forth.[35] Zichan discussed the background so extensively that such talk overshadowed his prognosis of the patient. Given such an emphasis, Zichan's knowledge of the spirits was hardly incidental. In other words, Zichan was no naturalist or "Confucian" humanist but rather a figure with essential knowledge of the spirits.

Other episodes in the *Tradition of Zuo* lend support to the view that the chroniclers depicted Attendant He's double (Zichan) as an expert on the spirits. When the people of Zheng experienced nightmares after the murder of a nobleman ousted from court, Zichan discerned the spiritual roots of the crisis. Taking his cues from the dreams, Zichan realized that the spirit of the murdered man was restless and would continue to haunt the living unless placated. Accordingly, Zichan reinstated the son of the murdered man, who had been stripped of rank and fortune in the aftermath of the murder. More importantly, Zichan allowed this son to offer sacrifices to the spirit of the murdered father, and so the nightmares ceased.[36]

A second episode involving the same Lord Ping provides an additional example of Zichan's prowess at interpreting signs from the numinous realm. Several years after the visit of Attendant He, Lord Ping became deranged and was confined to bed. By this time, Minister Zhao had died, and a new man had assumed a leading role in the governance of the state. This new minister dreamt about a golden bear entering the door of the lord's bedchamber. Suspecting that the bear was responsible for the illness, the minister asked Zichan, "What demon might this be?" This time, Zichan did not deny that spiritual forces were at work. The bear, Zichan told the minister, was a spirit to whom previous rulers of the state had offered sacrifices. So, Zichan inquired whether the Jin state ruler might have neglected the cult of the spirit. Being a man of superior judgment, the minister recognized the value of Zichan's advice and restored the sacrifices to the spirit. Not long afterward, the sick lord made a full recovery.[37]

An analysis of the text's structure thus discloses that Attendant He represented the textual double of Zichan. This is apparent from the similarities between the two figures: their positions within the narrative, the contents of their speeches, and their putative realms of expertise. The symmetry between the two episodes not only indicates that the chronicler exercised a high level of artistic license, but also that he added Attendant He for rhetorical effect. As a result, Attendant He looks more like a literary device rather than the historical figure behind a scientific revolution.

PERSONIFICATION OF AN ARCHETYPE

So far we have demonstrated that the chroniclers associated Attendant He not only with prophecies, but also with famous experts on the spirits. Yet this leaves another question: why would the chronicler show the healer both contradicting the diviners' conclusions and issuing a prophecy? To answer this question, it is necessary to look at the larger corpus of early narratives about medical divination and to ask whether Attendant He's speech fit a pattern. As revealed in the following text, a final reason exists to question the episode's historicity. Attendant He's denial of spiritual involvement conformed to an established archetype, namely, the expert of the numinous realm.

Before going further, it is worth noting that the chronicler did not treat all experts on the numinous realm equally. As Marc Kalinowski points out, there was a world of difference in the *Tradition of Zuo* between the diviners at court, on the one hand, and noblemen known for their understanding of spirits, on the other. The chronicler rarely associated diviners with any special discernment or knowledge of the numinous realm. In contrast, the same chronicler linked wise ministers and rulers, or noble experts, to more unconventional interpretations of the spirits and gods. When called upon to interpret dreams or omens, such noblemen challenged the interpretations of diviners and the necessity of offering sacrifices.[38]

The case of the southern Chu 楚 state king (fl. 489 BC) reveals that Attendant He's denial of spiritual involvement had parallels (see Table 1, #13).[39] According to the *Tradition of Zuo*, when the king fell ill, a divination was performed, and the Yellow River was named as the source. Interestingly, the king did not act on the information furnished by the diviner, prompting the nobles to request permission to offer sacrifices on the king's behalf. The king nevertheless resisted the pressure, explaining that the Yellow River lay beyond Chu borders, and so the river spirits did not have dominion over the king's realm (see Figure 3). Because of this, the king deemed it improper for him to sacrifice to these spirits. "According to the sacrificial mandates of the three dynasties of antiquity," he said, "the ruler should not make offerings that extend beyond the hills and mountains that can be seen from within the distance of the state."[40]

If one momentarily steps back from the specifics of the case, the commonalities with the illness of Lord Ping become apparent. To begin with, the chronicler depicted a familiar contest between the diviners and noble expert. Like Attendant He and his double, the king rejected the conclusions drawn from the divination. While he did not reveal the actual source of his illness, the king insisted that the results of the divination were misleading. The rejection of the diviner's conclusions did not amount, moreover, to doubt regarding the existence of the numinous realm. If anything, the king confirmed the power of the gods and the sacrificial obligations of human princes.

Table 1 *Records of Medical Divinations*

No	Date	Sick Person	Textual Source(s)
1	634 BC	Xiong Zhi 熊摯 of Kui 夔	*Zuozhuan* [Xi 26]
2	632	Lord of Jin	*Zuozhuan* [Xi 28]
3	609	Lord of Qi	*Zuozhuan* [Wen 18]
4	563	Lord of Jin	*Zuozhuan* [Xiang 10]
5	545	Mother of Wuyu 無宇	*Zuozhuan* [Xiang 28]
6	541	Lord Ping of Jin	*Zuozhuan* [Zhao 1]; *Guoyu* [Jinyu 8]
7	535	Lord Ping of Jin	*Zuozhuan* [Zhao 7]; *Guoyu* [Jinyu 8].
8	522	Lord Jing 景 of Qi	*Zuozhuan* [Zhao 20]; *Yanzi chunqiu* [*wai*], 7/3b–4b; *Yanzi chunqiu* [*nei*], 1/7b–8a; *Shanghai bowuguan*, VI: 159–91
9		Lord Jing of Qi	*Yanzi chunqiu* [*nei*], 6/2b–3a
10		Lord Jing of Qi	*Yanzi chunqiu* [*nei*], 3/5b–6a
11	516	Shusun Zhaozi 叔孫昭子 of Lu (the agent of his sudden death)	*Zuozhuan* [Zhao 26]
12	489	King Zhao 昭 of Chu	*Zuozhuan* [Ai 6]
13	489	King Zhao of Chu	*Zuozhuan* [Ai 6]
14	Ca. 431–407	King Jian 柬 of Chu	*Shanghai bowuguan*, v. 4, 195–215
15		King of Zhou	*Zhanguo ce*, 1/6a

Narratives that feature a nobleman who contested the results of a divination or argued against the necessity of performing sacrifices were not unique to the *Tradition of Zuo*. Similar themes run through historical chronicles and excavated manuscripts of roughly contemporaneous or later date, including the *Spring and Autumn Annals of Master Yan* (*Yanzi chunqiu* 晏子春秋) (see Table 1).

According to the *Annals of Master Yan*, there was nothing unusual about Attendant He disregarding the results of a divination and discussing heavenly retribution in the same breath. The best known of such episodes recounts the fever of the lord of Qi, which was interpreted by a famous minister by the name of Yan Ying 晏嬰 (d. 500 BC) (Table 1, #8).[41] By one account, this lord had been ill for more than a year. Confident that doubling the number of sacrifices would relieve him of illness, the lord dispatched two diviners to make rich offerings to the ancestral spirits – above and beyond what had been offered by his predecessors. Yet the lord's condition did not improve. Suspecting his diviners of foul play, the sick lord convened a meeting with several nobles including Yan Ying, announcing his plan to kill the diviners to appease the gods and to end the sickness. Predictably, the plan met with approval from the sycophants, but Yan Ying remained silent. Sensing opposition, the lord pressed Yan Ying for an answer, thus giving the minister an opening to express his disapproval. "Does Your Lordship," Yan Ying asked, "believe that offering prayers will bring benefits?" The lord responded affirmatively, prompting Yan Ying to say, "If this is the case, then cursing will also bring harm to Your Lordship." Yan Ying then explained how the lord's conduct invited the curses of the masses: the lord had overlooked wise ministers in favor of evil favorites. So the resentful commoners cursed the lord to heaven. If the whole state cursed the lord, Yan Ying added, there would be nothing that his diviners or their sacrifices could do to counteract the curses.[42]

Although the particulars were different, a number of parallels exist between this episode and Attendant He's visit to Jin. In contrast to Attendant He, Yan Ying did not question whether the illness had a spiritual root. Instead, Yan doubted that the deities were displeased for want of sacrifices. Still, the narrative is similar enough to the illness of Lord Ping. To begin with, the chief protagonist once more questioned the sacrificial logic of illness. Attendant He's rejection of spiritual causes opposed the idea that sacrifices of appeasement would always resolve illnesses. Yan Ying's position similarly overturned the simple arithmetic of sacrifice (i.e., the more sacrifices and prayers, the less susceptible the prince to illness). At the same time, neither of these figures denied the existence of gods or spirits. On the contrary, Yan affirmed the power of gods to make humans sick, and indeed, his sacrificial stance revealed a belief in Heavenly justice. Just as Attendant He stressed the power of Heaven to strike down negligent ministers, Yan Ying highlighted the connection between the conduct of the prince and his health. As Yan explained it to the lord, the only way to reverse the effects of the curse was to address the root problem: the quality of the lord's governance. If the lord ruled in a benevolent fashion and led an austere life, the collective curses would end, and the illness would improve.

A story about the illness of another Chu king comes still closer to articulating the positions found in the episode about Attendant He's visit to Jin. This story is preserved in a manuscript dating to the third or fourth century BC, which had been looted from a tomb before being bought from an auction by the Shanghai museum (Table 1, #14).[43] Possessing no known parallels in sources transmitted through the ages, this manuscript recounts a series of divinations performed in the Chu court in the fifth century BC, and the story goes as follows:

The king had fallen ill after observing a divination done to determine the cause of a long drought. The king subsequently dreamt of hills and streams and suspected that the nature spirits of a state recently annexed by Chu were responsible. As a result, the tortoise shell was consulted, but the nobles at court debated about what to do. One argued that the divination confirmed the correctness of the king's dream. The culprits were indeed the nature spirits of the new acquisition, so a sacrifice had to be made to appease them. Another noble, however, disagreed on the grounds of precedent; the earlier Chu kings, this noble reminded the other, had not offered sacrifices to the spirits in question, and so it was improper for the king to do so. At a loss about what to do, the pair consulted a third nobleman, described as a sage. The sage sided with the second noble, arguing that the spirits would reward the king for putting ancestral traditions above his health. "The ghosts, spirits, and the Lord-on-High [i.e., a god]," the sage explained, "are the most exalted and clear-sighted and so they invariably will know about the king's choice." "The king's illness," he furthermore promised, "will come to an end starting today."[44]

By now, all this should be familiar, because the Shanghai manuscript contains echoes of the episode about Lord Ping's illness. Much like Attendant He and Zichan, the sage challenged the conventional interpretation of the dream and divination (i.e., that offering sacrifices would placate the angry gods). At the same time, the sage affirmed the existence and power of the numinous realm, and in a later episode recounted in the same manuscript, the sage called for a sacrifice to be carried out by the king in order to end the drought. In this way, the sage affirmed the power of the spirits. Like Attendant He, he claimed that the spirits not only watched how men behaved but also rewarded or punished them.

By situating the figure of Attendant He within the larger corpus of divination narratives, one arrives at a third reason to question whether the figure's presentation in the *Tradition of Zuo* was historical. As shown in the preceding text, the fact that Attendant He rejected the results garnered through divination in one case and issued a prophecy about divine retribution in another was hardly strange. Such behavior was consistent with the tropes found in the larger corpus of historical chronicles, in which contested divinations and disputed sacrifices represented a leitmotif.

ATTENDANT HE AFTER THE TRADITION

A second look at the episode long regarded as "China's first medical case history" provides a new perspective on Attendant He. If one examines the narrative structure and discursive context with care, it becomes clear that the figure in the *Tradition of Zuo* did not occupy an important role in the medical tradition because of new or revolutionary ideas. The contributions of the original Attendant He, if he ever existed, are lost to us. Instead, the figure found in this text was a fictional persona that functioned primarily as a rhetorical device. Within that text, Attendant He personified an existing archetype. For this reason, it is unlikely that the views ascribed to the persona tell us much about the beliefs of healers during the Warring States period. On the contrary, I would argue that such views reflect the attitudes of chroniclers and their rhetorical conventions.

The later *Discourses of the States* (*Guoyu* 國語; comp. ca. late fourth–second century BC) further supports our reading of Attendant He. Although it resembles the episode in the *Tradition of Zuo*,[45] this later account furnishes a few new details. For a start, this later author dropped the theory of the six *qi* altogether and instead focused on Minister Zhao's impending death. As a result, the author reinforced the association between Attendant He and views of sickness and death as divine punishment. Moreover, the author added a telling remark not found in the earlier chronicle. At one point, Minister Zhao asked Attendant He whether the healer had a role to play in state affairs, to which the latter remarked, "The superior attendant rescues the state, whereas the inferior one merely attends to the sick person."[46] The healer's reported comment thus underscored the rhetorical interchangeability of the good minister and exemplary healer in early Chinese chronicles. It thus lends credibility to the proposition that the Attendant He found in the *Tradition of Zuo* was not a historical man, but a contrived rhetorical device.

Although the episode in the *Tradition of Zuo* was originally about something other than medicine, this fact was conveniently forgotten by later authors of medical treatises and histories.[47] One sixteenth-century work, the *History of Medicine* (*Yi shi* 醫史), provides a case in point. Its author even discussed how Attendant He discovered that the chief minister would die through an examination of the Lord of Jin. In the margins, this author noted that some were skeptical about the episode. To refute the skeptics' arguments, he recalled a controversy surrounding a Buddhist monk of the Song dynasty (AD 960–1279). The monk had been famous for his ability "to determine the station, luck, and virtues of a person based on an examination of the pulse." And like a divine being, the same monk told the fortune of a son based on the condition of the father.[48] This monk's penchant for fortune-telling had created a stir, with at least one famous man objecting that the monk's feats had no precedent in antiquity. Yet the famous minister Wang Anshi 王安石 (AD 1021–86) demurred, citing the example of Attendant He. "In ancient times," Wang said with approval, "Attendant He examined the pulse of the lord of Jin and determined that the lord's great minister was about to die." This led him to conclude, "If the fate of a minister can be seen in the pulse of the lord, what is so strange about a healer seeing the father and knowing the fate of the son?"[49]

The discussion in the Ming history of medicine is arresting for several reasons. For a start, it reveals that Attendant He's premodern reputation was different from his modern one. As we saw at the beginning, modern scholars nowadays characterize Attendant He as a great innovator in Chinese medical history – as China's first "naturalist," the healer had supposedly rejected demonic and spiritual explanations of illness. Although the sixteenth-century author also extolled Attendant He, he did so for reasons different from modern scholars. For this author, the ancient figure's fame owed much to his knowledge about matters other than illness. Instead, Attendant He stood apart from the others because of his ability to discern the will of Heaven and to foretell the future.

Differences aside, a single assumption unites both ancient and modern interpretations of the episode: namely, the belief that the *Tradition of Zuo* set forth an authoritative account of medical happenings. But where did this assumption come from? To answer this question, one must trace the process by which political parables came to be read as literal pieces of medical history.

2

BIAN QUE AS A SEER: POLITICAL PERSUADERS AND THE MEDICAL IMAGINATION

CHAPTER I SHOWED THAT, THOUGH REGARDED TODAY AS a source of ancient medical practice, the episode in the *Tradition of Zuo* was originally a political parable. For this reason, it would be ill-advised to treat the episode as a factual account of medical reasoning in early China. Yet this raises the question as to whether the case of Attendant He was an anomaly. To what extent did parties other than healers create representations of the medical fathers?

For answers, we are best served by turning to a famous story about another father of medicine: Bian Que's encounter with a stubborn patient. The story goes as follows: at a court audience, the famed healer warned a Lord Huan 桓 of a deadly ailment lodged between the lord's skin and flesh. As he was feeling well at the time, the lord scoffed. "You healers," the lord said with disdain, "like to treat those without sickness in order to accrue merit." Undeterred, Bian Que returned to repeat his warnings some days later, only to be ignored. The healer nevertheless came back for two more audiences, meeting a chillier reception each time. Not one to take a hint, Bian Que persisted in delivering his bad news, announcing that the illness had penetrated further into the lord's body. The lord, the healer pleaded, had to take action against the illness immediately, before it was too late. Bian Que's pleas fell on deaf ears. Several days after the final visit, the lord began to feel unwell and sent for the healer. Yet, by then Bian Que had fled the state, so the lord met his end.[1]

Unlike Attendant He, Bian Que is generally regarded by modern scholars as a mythical, rather than historical, figure. Pointing to one early pictorial representation of him, they argue that the figure had originally been a deity, a winged bird with a human head who subsequently became the patron god of healing.[2] In addition, a biography of Bian Que, compiled in the early first century BC, contains a number of implausible elements. If one trusts the biography, the famous encounter between Bian Que and Lord Huan would have occurred around 685 BC (earlier still, if one follows the dates implied by the version in another source) – in any event, almost *four* centuries before Bian Que's last recorded consultation with a patient.[3] Making matters worse, the historian tells us that Bian Que began practicing the curative arts only after drinking a magical potion that gave him the power to see through solid objects.[4]

Despite persistent questions about Bian Que's historicity, scholars have long assumed that the story offers a mirror of medical practice.[5] As Yamada Keiji puts it, the episode "presents a clear description of conceptions of illness and treatment" in the late Warring States (ca. 453–221 BC).[6]

But does the anecdote really tell us much about healers or healing during the Warring States? After all, the episode is recounted first *not* in a medical treatise but in a classic of statecraft, *Master Han Fei* (*Han Fei zi* 韓非子; comp. third century BC). Moreover, the main objective of *Master Han Fei* was not to explain medical theory and practice. Instead, the very titles of the chapters – for example, "The Way of the Ruler," "Wielding Power," "Precautions within the Palace," "The Eight Villainies," and the "Difficulties of Persuasion" – speak to the author's overriding interest in statecraft.

An additional reason exists to wonder whether the anecdote tells us much about medical practice or theory in the third century BC. As historian Han Jianping 韓健平 points out in a recent article, like most heroes of oral tradition, Bian Que was a malleable figure. If generations of storytellers remade this figure according to their aims and tastes, then one wonders how much of Bian Que – and the picture of medical practice associated with him – was created by persuaders such as Han Fei 韓非 (d. 233 BC), for whom this classic of statecraft was named.[7]

Through a close reading of the episode in *Master Han Fei*, the following discussion complements the findings of Chapter 1 by furthering our discussion of the contexts in which representations of exemplary healers were produced. At the same time, the present discussion goes beyond the previous chapter by addressing the relationship between those representations and medical theory. The discussion not only shows the dialectical relationship between the two domains of knowledge, but also illuminates the ways in which persuaders shaped the image of the medical fathers by reconfiguring aspects of medical practice.

My discussion opens by setting the stage: explaining the nature of our sources, as well as their historical backdrop. With such an introduction,

I turn to an analysis of our sources. I begin by revisiting assumptions about the encounter between Lord Huan and Bian Que, questioning whether the image of the healer was influenced by medical practice or by popular representations of the curative arts in the time of *Master Han Fei*. After considering these possibilities, I propose an explanation that fits better with the current body of evidence: while the episode in *Master Han Fei* drew upon elements of medical theory in the Warring States period, the image of Bian Que was also driven by the persuader's rhetorical goals and choice of metaphor. In particular, the persuader's habit of analogizing the healer to the sagacious minister prompted Bian Que's transformation into a figure who detected illnesses that eluded the sufferer. Viewed from this perspective, the iconic image of Bian Que was the product of persuaders, whose main objective was to stress the importance of preventive action in politics rather than to set forth a model of therapy.

SETTING THE STAGE

As much of our discussion revolves around the motives of Warring States persuaders, it would be useful to say something more about the period. Although the name derives from the protracted and increasingly large scale of its conflicts, the Warring States is also notable for its political breakthroughs, which represented the culmination of long historical processes that began in the sixth century BC. From that time, we see the rise of regimes headed by ruthless lords and ambitious advisors, which began supplanting the Spring and Autumn order. With these new regimes came more efficient systems of counting people and extracting resources, new modes of warfare, and higher technology. If the history of any one state were to epitomize this story, it would be Attendant He's home state of Qin, which rose to prominence in the fourth century BC and conquered much of what is now China in 221 BC. (For a map of the era, see Figure 6.)

The nature of our sources also bears clarification, being not only different in tenor from those seen in the previous discussion but also more varied in genre. In contrast to those of Chapter 1, our sources, composed of manuscripts recovered by archaeologists from tombs and deposits, actually address the nitty-gritty of medical practice and theory (see Table 2). These include the published contents of three sets of substantial manuscripts from the third and early second centuries BC, as well as a number of smaller fragments.[8]

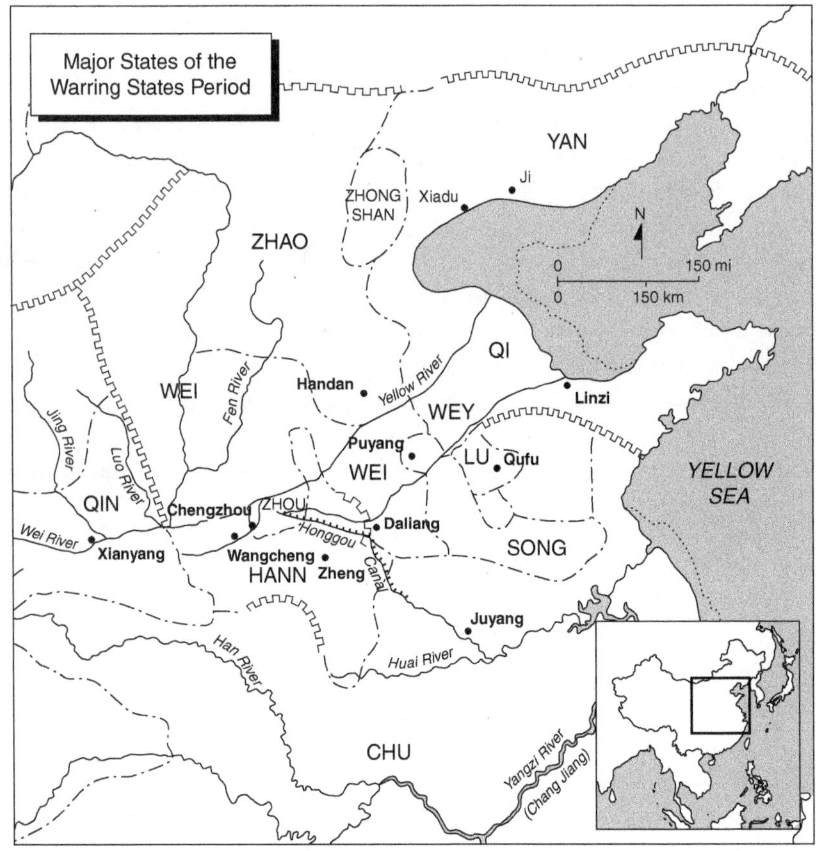

Figure 6 Map of the Warring States period, ca. 453–221 BC.

Source: *The Cambridge History of Ancient China: From the Origins of Civilization to 221 BC*, edited by Michael Loewe and Edward L. Shaughnessy (1999), 594. Reproduced with permission from Cambridge University Press.

In addition, the discussion incorporates classics of statecraft by persuaders (see Table 3). By persuaders, I mean the itinerant thinkers who traveled between the various political centers of preimperial and early imperial China, searching for patronage and ministerial positions. Such persuaders often made their cases to a ruler in person, delivering their policy recommendations in an oratorical fashion. Given these circumstances, it is unsurprising that the persuaders would have relied upon colorful historical anecdotes to hold the attention of potential patrons, including ones about legendary figures like Bian Que. Like chroniclers, the persuaders often preferred to narrate the events of earlier ages,

Table 2 *Excavated Medical Manuscripts Cited in This Chapter*

Name of Ms.	Date	Location
Guanju 關沮 formulas	209–206 BC	Guanju, Zhoujiatai 周家台 (South Central China)
Vessel Book (*Maishu* 脈書)	Third century BC	Zhangjiashan 張家山 (ca. 186 BC) and Mawangdui 馬王堆 (ca. 168 BC) (both South Central China)
Pulling Book (*Yinshu* 引書)	Uncertain; no later than 186 BC	Zhangjiashan (ca. 186 BC)
Methods for the Treatment of the Fifty-Two Illnesses (*Wushi'er bingfang* 五十二病方)	Before 168 BC	Mawangdui
Wuwei 武威 formulas and misc.	Early first century AD	Wuwei (NW China)

Table 3 *Classics of Persuasion Discussed in This Chapter*

Title	Approximate Date
Master Mo (*Mozi* 墨子)	Fourth to third century BC
Mencius (*Mengzi* 孟子)	Fourth to third century BC
Master Shi (*Shizi* 尸子)	Third century BC
Master of the Pheasant Cap (*Heguanzi* 鶡冠子)	Third century BC
Annals of Lü Buwei (*Lüshi chunqiu* 呂氏春秋	Comp. ca. 239 BC
Master Han Fei (*Han Fei zi* 韓非子)	Comp. ca. 233 BC

particularly those of the Spring and Autumn. By the same token, it also makes sense that the persuaders employed carefully chosen *analogies*, particularly when dealing with delicate subjects that might offend noble sensibilities – for example, the necessity of abandoning a life of pleasure and heeding the advice of wise ministers.

Some of the most famous persuaders include thinkers often referred to as philosophers: Mencius 孟子 (ca. 372–289 BC), Mo Di 墨翟 (ca. 479–381 BC), and Han Fei.[9] In general, persuaders focused in their writings on the critical role of the chief minister, a position to which they presumably aspired. In some of the cases discussed in the following text, a work of statecraft took its name from a persuader, a decision that reflected the fact that the persuader or his followers left behind treatises addressed directly to potential patrons.[10] In other cases, a work of several essays was named after a legendary minister idolized by the persuader, such as

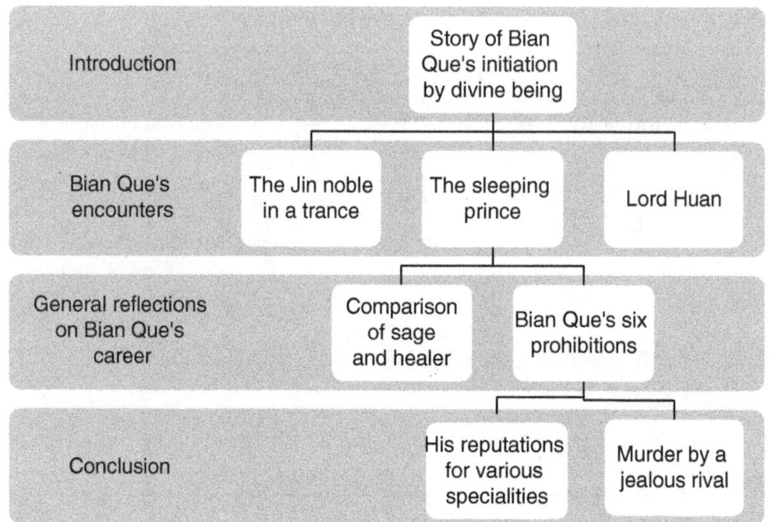

Figure 7 Biography of Bian Que at a glance. The figure shows the main elements of Sima Qian's biography in the *Records of the Grand Historian* (ca. 90 BC). Sima Qian drew many of these elements from existing sources, including Warring States–era classics of persuasion.

Source: Image drawn by author.

Shi Jiao 尸佼 (ca. 390–30 BC), an advisor to the famous Prime Minister Shang Yang 商鞅 (390–38 BC) in the state of Chu; or Guan Zhong 管仲 (d. ca. 645 BC), the chief counselor in the powerful state of Qi.

The *Records of the Grand Historian*, a chronicle attributed to the court scribe Sima Tan 司馬談 (fl. ca. 140–110 BC) and his son Sima Qian 司馬遷 (fl. ca. 140–86 BC), represents our final source. Completed around 90 BC, the *Records of the Grand Historian* is generally treated by scholars as the work of Sima Qian, and it encapsulates a wide range of subjects: the lives of mythical figures, the fortunes of noble houses and dynasties, persuaders, diviners, and political events in the Han court. One part of this monumental work concerns us in the following text, the first half of the "Biographies of Bian Que and the Granary Master" (*Bian Que Canggong liezhuan* 扁鵲倉公列傳).

As the second half of the joint biographies will be treated in subsequent chapters of this book, my remarks are restricted to the portion about Bian Que (see Figure 7). This portion, in four parts, opens with a tale about Bian Que's origins and the circumstances surrounding his initiation into the curative arts. The second part describes three encounters between Bian Que and patients. These include his visit to the state of Jin, which was under the stewardship of a powerful noble who had fallen into a trance; Bian Que's miraculous revival of a sick prince (see Chapter 3); and finally, the aforementioned encounter with Lord Huan. The third part offers general reflections about Bian Que's career: the sagacious qualities of the healer, and the six prohibitions attributed to him, or the six conditions in which healers were not to treat patients. The fourth and final part explains Bian Que's reputation as a master healer of various sorts, his murder at the hands of an assassin, and the fact that the legendary figure was synonymous with the art of the pulse in the historian's time.

One aspect of Sima Qian's practice of historical writing bears explanation, and we will return to this point repeatedly. A veritable *bricoleur*, Sima fashioned his biography of Bian Que largely out of recycled textual material, stitched together from passages drawn from classics of statecraft and older historical chronicles. Consider the three descriptions of Bian Que's encounters with patients. As we have already seen, the episode about Lord Huan was probably drawn from *Master Han Fei*, as Sima Qian was familiar with the text, having used large portions of it to compose his portrait of the persuader.[11] Similarly, Sima Qian must have lifted the second episode involving the sleeping prince from classics of statecraft, as this story surfaces in later works of that genre.[12] The provenance of the last of the episodes is less clear-cut, due to the lack of attested parallels in extant documents. Even so, the evidence suggests that Sima Qian did *not* create the story from thin air. The story resembles the episode in the *Tradition of Zuo*, discussed in Chapter 1, which suggests that Sima Qian appropriated it from an existing chronicle.[13]

As we shall see, Sima Qian had at his disposal a rich body of lore to create his image of the iconic figure. Like the persuaders and chroniclers before him, Sima Qian would exploit that lore to further his rhetorical goals in the chapter. Yet before we can say anything about Sima Qian's role in creating the modern image of the famed healer, we must know something more about the historian's sources: who created them and to what end?

MIRROR OF CONTEMPORARY HEALING?

I have already mentioned that Yamada and other modern scholars take for granted that the episode about Bian Que reflected medical thinking in the third century BC, but is such an assumption warranted? To answer this question, the central premise of *Master Han Fei* – to wit, that healers sought to detect *and* treat illnesses before the sufferer ailed – must be interrogated. As we shall see, this philosophy of treatment is missing from surviving medical works that circulated around the time of Master Han Fei. Though common elements exist, these contemporary works are unlike *Master Han Fei* insofar as they emphasize tangible and obvious symptoms in patients. As a result, the episode should *not* be regarded as a transcription of the curative arts in the author's time.

The earliest surviving medical manuscripts, which archaeologists have recovered from the Guanju 關沮 site (ca. 209–206 BC), offer no hint that illnesses could be treated in advance of discomfort or noticeable symptoms.[14] Instead, the authors of these manuscripts focused on illnesses that presented themselves through obvious, serious, and extraordinary symptoms. If such authors believed that someone could be sick even if he or she appeared or felt well (as was the case with Lord Huan), they never mentioned this possibility. Consider the following entry, which is representative of the manuscript as a whole. The author explained what to do in cases in which there is a lump in the abdomen. "Burn a sword with a square end," the authors wrote, "tempering it by dipping it in fine liquor; women should use it twice seven times, and men seven times." If this is done, the author added, the lump will disappear.[15]

Judging from the rest of the manuscript, the silence about anything other than full-blown or obvious ills was not accidental, but rather reflected a larger pattern where illnesses were defined by their symptoms. This pattern can be gleaned from the nature of the ailments discussed in the manuscript, which are largely synonymous with the symptoms. These include fevers and chills (*nüe* 瘧), warm disorders (*wenbing* 瘟病), ascending *qi*, heat disorders (*dan* 單 or *danbing* 憚病), moles or birthmarks (*heizi* 黑子), atrophy (*weibing* 痿病), abscesses (*yong* 癰), ailments affecting the heart such as lumps (*jiaxin ji* 瘕心疾), and tooth decay (the last of which received its share of attention).

Surely, too much can be made of the discrepancies between *Master Han Fei* and the earliest medical manuscripts. After all, considerations of genre need to be taken into account. Formula books like that found at the Guanju site were arguably for self-treatment rather than for trained healers like Bian Que. In other words, the authors of such books did *not* assume much by way of specialized training or knowledge. Thus, one would expect that the text would stick to illnesses that required no telling touch or trained eye to detect. And indeed, a similar view of diagnosis is found in other manuscripts designed for self-treatment, particularly those discovered at the Mawangdui 馬王堆 site[16] (which probably dates to the late third century BC).[17] The *Treatment of the Fifty-Two Illnesses* (*Wushi'er bingfang* 五十二病方), for example, features ailments marked by conspicuous symptoms: distended bellies, inguinal swellings, and wounds from metal objects. Other entries in the same manuscript point to signs including warts, pimples, and "facial pustules" with bursting abscesses. Naturally, the ailments did not have to be visible to the external observer to be obvious or grotesque to the afflicted. A large number of them, in fact, were located in the nether regions. For example, the author devoted considerable space on the many varieties of hemorrhoids (the most memorable of which were characterized by numerous openings, out of which crawled white pinworms).[18] Though out of sight, these ailments were no less obvious, because the discomfort announced that something was amiss. A later manuscript discovered at the northwestern frontier of Wuwei 武威 (first century AD), which is similar to the *Treatment of the Fifty-Two Illnesses* with respect to content and style, further suggests that the marked absence of the kinds of illnesses described in *Master Han Fei* owed much to differences between genres.[19] The manuscript also focused on afflictions synonymous with the symptoms: persistent coughs accompanied by wheezing, abdominal swellings, feelings of internal coldness, problems with impotence, and the appearance of swollen scrotums that oozed from the base a yellow juice.[20]

Though worth bearing in mind, the discrepancies between *Master Han Fei* and contemporary medical texts should not simply be chalked up to genre. Archaeologists have also discovered manuals for diagnosing vessel illnesses (*maishu* 脈書), one of which was buried with a formula book in the same tomb. These manuals, moreover, were arguably *not* for self-treatment; they supplied instructions for diagnosing ills in cases in which the sick person had gone mad or had lost his wits. Consider, for example, the following excerpt from a manual unearthed at the Zhangjiashan 張家山 site (ca. 186 BC), which provides directions for determining the source of an illness:

> 是 勭(動)即病, 悒悒如亂, 坐而起, 則目 晾 如無見, 心如縣(懸), 病饑, 氣不足, 善怒, 心狄(惕)狄(惕) , 恐人將捕之, 不欲食, 面黯若灺色, 欬(咳)則有血, 此為骨蹶(厥), 是少陰之脈主治。

> If the vessel is agitated, then there will be an illness. The person will be dejected as if he is disordered. When he rises from a seated position, his eyes will go dark as if he cannot see. The heart will be as if suspended, and the person will be afflicted from starvation and lacking in *qi*.[21] He will be prone to rage, and his heart will be terrified, as he will fear that

> someone is coming to capture him. He will not desire to eat anything, and his face will be as dark as the charcoal of extinguished candle drippings. When he coughs, there will be blood. This is due to bone reversal, and these illnesses can be controlled and treated at the site of the Lesser Yin vessel.[22]

What is evident from the excerpt – one of ten such descriptions in the manuscript – is the attention given to symptoms, concrete and obvious ones, at that. Such descriptions have a palpable, even visceral, feel to them: the color of the complexion, the clouding of the eyes as one rises, and the pangs of hunger or the marked absence of an appetite. In this passage, it is the patient's experience of illness, as Vivienne Lo points out, that serve as the focus in the diagnosis of ills.[23]

If contemporary medical texts failed to mention the treatment of ills before the onset of discomfort, then how does one account for the story about Lord Huan's illness? To put it baldly, should we consider the story a fanciful representation of medical practice? This scenario is worth considering, if only because *Master Han Fei* is a highly rhetorical text, and historians have voiced their suspicions regarding the historicity of the episode in question.[24] Such suspicions owe much to the fact that persuaders were notorious for their fictionalized retellings of the past. What is more, ancient men were hardly ignorant of the artistic license exercised by persuaders, something indicated by complaints about their penchant for "using the past to serve the present."[25] All this raises the following question: if court persuaders were comfortable embellishing, if not entirely reinventing, historical events to convey their own political messages, then what was to stop them from altering the picture of medical practice, too?

Although it was not a transcription of common medical practices, the story should not be dismissed as pure fiction either. The very fact that *Master Han Fei* could use the encounter between Bian Que and Lord Huan in a rhetorical fashion implied some common core of beliefs about the body. Without these beliefs, the encounter would have been meaningless. Because of this, it is worth considering whether the story was based at least *loosely* on elements of curative practice, elements that would have been recognizable to the audience.

If one adopts a looser standard of evidence, the connection between early medical texts and *Master Han Fei* becomes more apparent. In surviving medical treatises of that era, one finds the isolated elements of the Bian Que episode scattered between different manuscripts: for example, the idea that someone could diagnose an illness without the patient's input, as well as the notion that it was possible to forestall pain or deadly ailments.[26]

The authors of surviving manuals *did* hint that it was possible for a healer like Bian Que to diagnose an illness that eluded the sick person's detection. Consider, for example, the following instructions for determining the source of an illness *just* by palpating the ankle:

> 它脈盈, 此獨虛, 則主病。它脈滑, 此獨㴩 (澀), 則主病。它脈靜, 此獨 𨔼 (動), 則主病。夫脈固有𨔼 (動)者, 骭之少陰, 臂之鉅陰、少陰, 是主𨔼 (動), 疾則病。此所以論有過之脈殹 (也)。

> If the pulse from the other vessels is full but this alone is empty, then this vessel is the host of the illness. If the other vessels are flowing smoothly but this one alone is rough, then this vessel is the host of the illness. If the other vessels are tranquil, and this one alone is agitated, the vessel is the host of the illness. As for the vessels that necessarily have pulsations, these include the Lesser Yin of the shin,[27] the Greater Yin of the forearm, and the Lesser Yin of the forearm. These control the pulsations (of the other vessels?). If the pulse is hurried, there is an illness in one of these vessels. This is the way to determine excess in the vessels.[28]

The passage provides a few points worth drawing out. Notice here that the author focused solely upon the quality of the pulse: rough, agitated, hurried, and tranquil. Unlike pain, none of these were signs accessible to the sick person; instead, the healer obtained them solely through examination. In addition, such signs were *subtle* cues in the pulse, cues unlike the very overt or grotesque symptoms described in previous excerpts. By mentioning faint bodily signs discernible only to the healer, the author implied that it was possible for someone to detect the presence of illness solely through the examination of the pulse. The sick person, in other words, did not necessarily have privileged knowledge of his or her body.

Theoretical possibilities aside, the author of the manual stopped short of saying that healers *actually* diagnosed sicknesses without consulting the ill. Indeed, the sheer amount of space given to obvious symptoms in the manuscript suggests the opposite: namely, that the author put greater weight on the subjective experience of the sick person over irregularities in the pulse (or, for that matter, subtle changes in the appearance).[29] The stress on obvious signs is also evident from the varying level of detail in the manuscript. There, the perfunctory, even impoverished, discussions of pulse diagnosis stand in relief to the rich and elaborate descriptions of symptoms associated with the same illnesses.

In addition, contemporary medical texts revealed an interest in prevention, one that resembled the idea of treating illnesses before the patient ailed. In this respect, the *Pulling Book* (*Yinshu* 引書) – which set forth directions for therapeutic stretches and breathing exercises – provides a prime example. Granted, the possibility that a person could unwittingly be sick never came up. If anything, such an idea was foreign to the author of the manuscript. Most of the illnesses in the text were marked by obvious signs of something amiss: back discomfort, knee pain, abdominal swelling, exhaustion, and so forth.[30] Even so, the *Pulling Book* did highlight the importance of preventing illness or prophylaxis – a notion that resembled Bian Que's purported insistence on early treatment. The text laid out regimens that harmonize the patterns of eating, sleeping, and sexual activity with the seasons. By the author's account, such regimens worked to shore up the body's store of vital essence and offered protection against illnesses resulting from the lack of harmony between the body and cosmic cycles.[31]

A survey of early Chinese medical texts has thus revealed that the diagnostic practices associated with Bian Que in *Master Han Fei* were neither a reflection of contemporary healing techniques nor a fanciful story. On the one hand, contemporary sources presented a different picture of therapy insofar as they stressed the patient's feelings of discomfort over subtle cues found in the appearance or pulse. Yet on the other hand, one finds elements of the story in various medical manuscripts. The emphasis on prevention in contemporary medical manuscripts, for instance, echoed Bian Que's calls for early treatment. In addition, the authors of manuals left open the possibility that it was at least theoretically possible for a healer to diagnose an illness in the absence of overt symptoms or discomfort. For all of these reasons, the episode in *Master Han Fei* was *not* a facsimile of contemporary medical practice; instead, it represented an imaginative reworking of elements drawn from medical manuscripts.

URBAN LEGEND?

So what inspired the portrait of Bian Que in *Master Han Fei*? One possibility, explored in the following text, is that the author of *Master Han Fei* drew upon existing legends of Bian Que or healers more generally. This explanation admittedly has its virtues. References to sickness are copious in historical chronicles and other works from preimperial China. As one scholar notes in her study of preimperial thought, the body provided a convenient metaphor for writers, who exploited its rhetorical potential.[32] By examining the preimperial corpus, our discussion reveals that while certain elements of Bian Que's encounter with Lord Huan were inspired by calls for timely intervention, there were also salient differences: the idea of treating illnesses in advance of discomfort was uncommon.

When set against the larger corpus of preimperial texts, the Bian Que found in *Master Han Fei* was largely unprecedented. Like the medical texts examined in the preceding discussion, most early representations of healing focus on acute or obvious cases of sickness. The *Tradition of Zuo*, which provides one of the most extensive records of illness with its forty-five cases of sickness, illustrates this point.[33] In this lengthy chronicle, references to latent ills that erupt suddenly and without warning are notably absent. The absence is striking considering the fact that the text contains references to sudden deaths "without illness." In one case, the chronicler claimed that a minister died while seeking to restore the fortunes of his state. Despite what one might expect, the chronicler accounted for the minister's death in terms of divine retribution rather than an illness of which the minster was unaware. According to the chronicler, Heaven had "forsaken" the state and was punishing its ruler by depriving him of a conscientious minister.[34]

Moreover, the earliest references to Bian Que associate him only with full-blown illnesses, not cases in which the person mistakenly believed that he or she was well. This is evident from the depiction of the famed healer in another chronicle, the *Stratagems of the Warring States* (*Zhanguo ce* 戰國策; third century BC?). In one episode, Bian Que is invoked to drive home the necessity of taking harsh remedies for obvious ailments like "swellings and abscesses."[35] Such a presentation is also evident in a second episode involving Bian Que's visit to the state of Qin. There, Bian Que had an audience with the king, who summoned the healer because he was feeling sick. In the audience, the healer proposed to rid the king of the illness, a proposal that met great opposition from the king's courtiers. "Your Majesty's illness," the courtiers told the king, "is located in the area in front of the ears and below the eyes." "If you try to get rid of it," they warned, "the illness will not necessarily be cured but you could lose the keenness of your ears and the clarity of your eyes." The king reported the comments to Bian Que, who angrily retorted, "If this is how the state of Qin is governed, then it will perish as soon as Your Majesty acts."[36] Several aspects of the episode invite comparison to the one in *Master Han Fei*. Unlike Lord Huan (another difficult patient), the king actually acknowledged that he was sick. The problem instead lay with the king's refusal to literally take the medicine. For Bian Que, such a refusal portended the political demise of Qin, for it revealed the king's unwillingness to employ tough – albeit necessary – measures to ensure the health of the state.

The focus on acute and obvious ailments represents a larger pattern in historical chronicles, including the *Discourses of the States* (see Chapter 1). The episode involving the invasion of Qi by a southern power, Wu 吳,[37] in the fifth century BC, presents a case in point. At the time, the ruler of the Yue 越, another power in the South, sent emissaries to the Wu court with bribes, which delighted the nobles in Wu to no end. Yet a more discerning member of the Wu court warned, "The presence of the Yue among us is like an illness of the heart and abdomen, as their territory is equal to ours but they nevertheless have designs on our land." The advisor then proposed to attack the Yue. Anticipating resistance, the advisor explained his reasoning through the following analogy: "One does not order a healer to remove an illness and then ask him to leave some of it behind."[38] In this case, the author did not characterize the threat posed by the Yue as an incipient ill. On the contrary, the wording here – note the reference to "removal" (*chu* 除), a turn of phrase that conjured up the removal of an ungainly growth – implied that the Yue was a clear and present danger.

Thus far, our discussion has been confined to chronicles, which stand apart from *Master Han Fei* in genre, but do precursors to the Bian Que episode exist in other works of persuasion? With its emphasis on timing, the *Master Mo* (*Mozi* 墨子; comp. ca. fourth to third century BC) resonates with some of the themes in *Master Han Fei*.[39] There, the author stated that using music and rites to bring order to a chaotic state is like "digging a well after one begins to hiccup" or "seeking a healer *after* the sick person has died." Interestingly, the author did not recommend treating the illness before the sick person experienced discomfort. True to his penchant for hammering the point home, the Mohist author instead chose to belabor the obvious. The reader was reminded that the healer (and thus his political analogue, the minister) should act *before* the illness completely ran its course and killed the patient.[40]

With its emphasis on timely intervention, the *Master Shi* (*Shizi* 尸子; third century BC) offers parallels to the description of Bian Que in *Master Han Fei*. To stress the importance of heeding the advice of wise ministers, *Master Shi* relates the allegory of a minister who wailed for three days. Someone had overheard the wailing and asked the minister about the reason for such a display of grief, to which the minister replied that his state was about to perish. The minister then went on to explain his reasons for believing that the end was imminent. "I have heard that when the sick person is about to die," he said, "it is impossible to be a good healer, just as when a state is about to perish, it is futile to make plans." "I have admonished my lord numerous times but to no avail," he added, "so this is how I know that the state is about to perish!"[41] Once more, the author employed the analogy between healer and minister to highlight the importance of timely action in politics. At the same time, there is one substantial difference here worth noting: unlike *Master Han Fei*, this classic of statecraft stopped short of claiming that ills could be treated *before* the onset of obvious symptoms.

THE SAGE AND THE HEALER

Many of the elements of Bian Que's encounter with Lord Huan had precedents in other sources and genres. Even so, there was a gap between the emphasis on timely or preventive care, on the one hand, and the specific call to treat illnesses before someone ailed, on the other. To explain how the gap was closed, it would be instructive to return to the episode in *Master Han Fei*. By examining it alongside other works that associate Bian Que with what the persuaders referred to as "ills that do not ail" (*bubing bing* 不病病), I show that the image of Bian Que in *Master Han Fei* was molded by its object of comparison, the prescient minister.

Let us begin with a discussion of the author's goals. If we look more closely at the larger context of the episode in *Master Han Fei*, it becomes clear that the author did not relate Bian Que's feats to illuminate the finer points of medical theory. As Yamada Keiji puts it, the author recited the anecdote to impress readers with a general point: the need to spot and root out political troubles while they are still "small," or before they become full-blown crises.[42] To this observation, I would also add that the episode illustrates the sage's ability to spot signs of trouble ahead of time. "Since the boundaries between fortune and calamity lie in the margin between the skin and flesh, the *sage* deals with trouble well in advance." In this text, the sage is not merely a wise or virtuous person, but a perspicacious figure. Like Sherlock Holmes, the sage can spot premonitions of trouble through small cues, or "tells." Or as *Master Han Fei* puts it, "The sage is one who sees the subtle and learns of the sprouts of things."[43]

Surely, too much can be made of the references to sages in *Master Han Fei*. Sages *were* hardly new or unique to third-century texts, raising the possibility that the focus on "ills that do not ail" had little to do with conceptions of sages at all. In fairness, the notion of perspicacity did predate the time of *Master Han Fei*.[44] A similar constellation of ideas, in fact, runs through historical chronicles like the *Tradition of Zuo*, where methods for divining the future based on body language are discussed. According to Marc Kalinowski, such methods involved making predictions about imminent events – for example, the downfall of a ruler or the decline of a state – based on the interpretation of tells: the hushed tone in which a man speaks, the posture of a ruler, and a person's lack of reverence in accepting offerings on ritual occasions.[45] Writing of these methods for divining the future, one Han dynasty social critic went so far as to argue that they inspired myths about the perspicacity of sages. As this man put it, "In the Spring and Autumn period (ca. 771–453 BC), the nobles and grandees would convene and observe changes in conduct, listen for talk of plots; if the signs were positive, they learned of portents of good fortune; but if bad, they learned of portents of disaster."[46]

Precursors notwithstanding, the image of the perspicacious sage emerged relatively late in the preimperial period. Although they highlighted the moral perceptiveness of such figures, earlier works did not ascribe any special prescience or perspicacity to sages. In fact, the *Mencius* (*Mengzi* 孟子; comp. fourth to third century BC) hinted that sages could be no more discerning of character than anyone else or necessarily capable of seeing through ruses. One of the greatest of all sages had even entrusted his brothers with territory, only to find himself betrayed when the brothers rebelled against the rightful king.

On the contrary, the perspicacity of sages became a motif in classics of persuasion *after* the third century BC, when the ability to anticipate trouble represented the litmus test of the sage. Such notions are elaborated in another classic of persuasion, the *Annals of Lü Buwei* (*Lüshi chunqiu* 呂氏春秋; comp. ca. 239 BC). In this work, the sage is credited with prescience with respect to rebellions, a quality the authors explained in terms of the sage's unusual ability to "scrutinize external signs and cues" in gestures likened to "autumn hairs," or described as "minutiae" and "subtleties."[47]

For a concrete sense of the sage's ability to detect signs of troubles to come, we turn to the description of the aforementioned minister, Master Guan, in the *Annals of Lü Buwei*. What follows in my discussion is but one of a collection of tales that extols the perspicacity of Master Guan, tales that highlight the minister's ability to interpret visual or aural clues in the deportment of people harboring secrets.[48] The tale goes as follows. Lord Huan and Master Guan had been plotting to attack the state of Ju 莒 before their plans became widely known. Taken aback by the leak, Master Guan remarked, "There must be a sage in the state." Lord Huan thereupon guessed that the sage was one of the workers outside of the palace. The next day, the pair summoned the worker and asked him how he knew about the planned attack. The worker answered that the gentleman had three kinds of expressions. One was of pleasure, befitting someone listening to music; the second was of sorrow, appropriate for someone wearing mourning; and the last was of anger, of someone about to go to war. The worker then explained how this related to his specific observations of the pair. He had seen the lord in a rage from the top of a terrace. "The movement of your lordship's hands and feet," the worker said, "were restrained – the appearance of someone about to go to war, and your lordship opened his mouth but did not close it." The worker had furthermore noticed that the lord was making the shape of "Ju" with his mouth. Because the lord raised his arm, the worker inferred that Lord Huan was preparing to go to war with the state of Ju.[49] In this episode, the ability to infer the hidden or formless from subtle cues was not something everyone was thought capable of. Instead, as the reactions of Master Guan revealed, the skill was unique to sages. As the author put it in the concluding remarks about the episode, "The sage hears that which is without sound and sees that which is without form."[50]

Thus far, I have situated Bian Que's encounter with Lord Huan within a larger discursive tradition about the perspicacity of sages, but I have yet to say anything about how exactly the healer's image was reshaped by its object of comparison. The link between the healer's image and the analogy is more explicit in another classic of statecraft, the *Master of the Pheasant Cap* (*Heguanzi* 鶡冠子; comp. ca. third century BC?),[51] in which Bian Que appears *not* as the ideal healer, but as the younger brother of one. In this connection, it would be useful to examine the conversation between a ruler and an advisor, in which a vignette about Bian Que and his brother is embedded. In conversation, the advisor affirmed the importance of finding sages, arguing that the rise of past powers owed much to perspicacious advisors who "attended" or "looked after the health" (*yi* 醫) of the heads of state. By way of illustration, the same advisor related an earlier dialogue between Bian Que and another ruler. Learning that Bian Que came from a family of three brothers, all of whom practiced medicine, the lord asked the famed healer which of the brothers possessed the best skills. A paragon of fraternal devotion, Bian Que answered that while he was the most famous, both of his elder brothers were superior to him in terms of ability: "My eldest brother can observe the illness while it is ethereal, and before it has taken shape, he has gotten rid of it." Though less accomplished than the first, his second brother was also more impressive than Bian Que, as this brother could "treat illnesses when they reside in the autumn's hairs (i.e., when the illness is infinitesimal)." Bian Que's powers of detection, in contrast, were limited, as he was capable of only detecting illnesses that exhibited full-blown symptoms and so had to make recourse to harsh remedies. The healer's comments made an impression on his noble interlocutor, who immediately seized upon the implications for statecraft: sagacious ministers like Master Guan treat ills before they become apparent, so as to avoid harsh remedies that damage the integrity of the body politic. Or, as the author explains, "In allowing Master Guan to 'attend to him' in the way of Bian Que, Lord Huan of Qi was indeed able to become overlord, because in all cases, the 'ills that do not ail' were treated before they had names and prevented from taking shape. . . ."[52]

The resonances between the *Master of the Pheasant Cap* and *Master Han Fei* are worth rehearsing, as they reveal how healers and the "ills that do not ail" represented the rhetorical double of sages and hidden political troubles. For a start, the emphasis here is on treating illnesses that do not already present a clear and present danger. According to the author, illnesses exist even before the sick experience discomfort. In their beginning stages, illnesses are ethereal but then become increasingly apparent over time, which brings us to an additional point: the importance of prophylaxis, as the goal is to avoid harsh remedies. What is more, the author recounts the story of Bian Que and his brother to illustrate the importance of employing sages, who deal with political crises before they get out of hand. Such sages are masters at deciphering early signs of treachery or deceit, and so they can root out troubles even before such problems take shape. In this case, the author compares Bian Que (or better still, his eldest brother) to a particular sage, Master Guan, a revealing comparison because the minister was the sage *par excellence*. As seen in the preceding text, Master Guan was credited by many persuaders with catapulting the state of Qi to a position of unrivaled power, because he detected plots before they could be carried out, thereby forestalling political crises.

When set against the broader tradition of the persuaders, it becomes clear that the specific call to treat the "ills that do not ail" within *Master Han Fei* owed much to rhetorical necessity. In this tradition, the figure of the healer stood in a metaphorical relationship to the minister. The persuaders furthermore likened the ills of the state to those of the body, with political crises such as invasions and rebellions serving as the analogues to swellings and pus. Accordingly, they analogized harsh measures to suppress political troubles to the healer's attempts to eliminate ills of the body. In the third century BC, however, the analogy was reconfigured in response to the new focus on the perspicacious sage. In this way, the "ills that do not ail" became a rhetorical double for hidden political threats, and the elimination of sickness before the onset of obvious symptoms a metaphor for measures to forestall political crises.

THE AFTERLIFE OF AN ANALOGY

Like Chapter 1, the preceding discussion reveals that someone other than healers created the representations of the medical fathers still used today as sources of early Chinese medical history. In the case of this iconic story about Bian Que, the key players were the persuaders of the Warring States rather than healers. By creatively adapting elements of medical practice and overlaying them on top of the archetype of the sagely minister, a stock figure in classics of statecraft, ancient persuaders created the perspicacious image of Bian Que. Such persuaders, I further show, crafted the image of the legendary figure *not* to expound on specific medical principles but to illustrate a political point.

So when did authors begin to treat the episode not as a political parable but as an actual historical event? The first sign of the episode being read in this way is relatively late, the *Records of the Grand Historian* of Sima Qian. At first glance, it would seem that Sima Qian did not add much to the account found in *Master Han Fei*. For the most part, the version in the *Records of the Grand Historian* represents a verbatim quotation from the earlier classic of statecraft. Even so, there are signs of Sima Qian's editorial discretion at work. To see this, one must remember that by the time Sima Qian compiled the *Records of the Grand Historian*, a wide array of stories about Bian Que had been circulating across various genres and works. But not all of these stories found their way into Sima Qian's biography of the figure. Consider the account of Bian Que's origins. As we have already seen, there was at least one tradition found in the corpus of the persuaders that claimed that the legendary figure hailed from a family of healers. Interestingly, Sima Qian did *not* repeat this account in his biography, choosing instead to relate the story of Bian Que's initiation into the arts by a mysterious being. According to Sima Qian, Bian Que had worked at a lodge house in his youth, where he met a mysterious guest. Impressed, the youth made every effort to become acquainted with the guest, described by Sima Qian as a divine being. After ten years of association, the divine being finally pulled Bian Que aside and bestowed a potion upon the young man, giving him the power to see through solid objects like walls and presumably human bodies.[53]

This was not the only way that Sima Qian crafted Bian Que's image; the historian also made subtle adjustments to the figures in the story. For example, *Master Han Fei* identified the patient in question as Lord Huan of the state of *Cai* 蔡 (ca. 714–695 BC). Sima Qian, in contrast, presented the patient as a lord of *Qi* by the same name (ca. 685–644 BC).[54] By adjusting the identity of Bian Que's patient, Sima Qian strengthened the analogy between the sagely minister and exemplary healer. Through these means, Bian Que's political counterpart became none other than Master Guan, who, as we already saw, was the epitome of the sagely minister.

Aside from introducing such small but telling changes, Sima Qian's reworking of existing materials also imparted new meanings to the encounter between Bian Que and Lord Huan, something revealed by the contrast between his remarks and those found in *Master Han Fei*. *Master Han Fei* drew out the following message about the importance of controlling political threats from the episode: "In treating ills, the good healer attacks while they reside in the space between the skin and flesh: this is to strike while the ills are still minute." *Master Han Fei* then concluded with the general reflection, "As the boundaries between fortune and calamity lie in the space between the skin and flesh, the *sage* deals with trouble well in advance."[55] The remarks in the *Records of the Grand Historian* were briefer: "Just as a sage is able to know things ahead of time because of his knowledge of the subtle, the good healer is able to act upon things in advance, and so illnesses can be done away with and the body revived."[56]

The concluding remarks on the episode are quite different. In *Master Han Fei*, the persuader started with what exemplary healers like Bian Que did, using it to illustrate the conduct of the sagely minister. In other words, the healer functioned as a political metaphor. In the *Records of the Grand Historian*, however, Sima Qian reversed the order of comparison. The discussion began with the conduct of sagely ministers, conduct that Sima Qian used to explain the achievements of exemplary healers like Bian Que. In other words, the political figure explicated the exemplary healer. The different uses of the analogy between the body and body politic paralleled the diverging goals between the texts. In *Master Han Fei*, the story about Bian Que's encounter with Lord Huan explained a key principle of statecraft: the importance of rooting out political threats before they became full blown. In the *Records of the Grand Historian*, in contrast, the same episode figured in a biographical narrative that elucidated the career of a famous figure, one removed from the original context of statecraft. By reconfiguring the existing analogy between minister and healer, Sima Qian found a novel way to read the episode.

Although it put a new spin on the anecdote, the biography of Bian Que did not represent a complete break with *Master Han Fei.* This biography also contained an element of allegory. As Jin Shiqi writes, the chapter in the *Records of the Grand Historian* was multivalent and thus should be read at different levels. Besides revealing the personal history of a famous figure, it also made a rhetorical point, one that depended on the existing analogy between healer and minister. When Sima Qian related how Bian Que was murdered by an assassin hired by an envious rival, one should not read the story merely as exposing the dangers that talented healers faced. Such a story also exposed the perils of political life, something hinted at in Sima Qian's final remarks about the disastrous consequences of attracting jealousy at court.[57]

While the allegorical dimensions of the biography must be kept in mind, the novelty of Sima Qian's interpretation of the encounter between Bian Que and Lord Huan deserves mention. By extracting earlier anecdotes about Bian Que from works of persuasion and explicit discussions of statecraft, Sima Qian wove together the various strands of legends and textual fragments in a narrative about the career and life of a healer. In so doing, he primed future readers to see the persuader's materials in a biographical light, paving the way for later interpretations of the episode as medical history.

Sima Qian was not alone in reinterpreting the stories told about Bian Que by persuaders. Medical texts a century after Sima Qian's time abounded with references to the virtues of treating incipient ills, or "ills that have yet to ail" (*weibing* 未病), a turn of phrase suggesting familiarity with the language of the persuaders.[58] For this, one only has to turn to the *Yellow Emperor's Inner Classic* (*Huangdi neijing* 黄帝内經; hereafter *Inner Classic*). Compiled more than two centuries after *Master Han Fei,* in the late first century BC or AD, the text presented the ideal healer as nothing less than a sage, a figure skilled at rooting out ills before they became serious. In this regard, it is worth noting the comments about one illness: "When it strikes people, the effects are subtle, and no one is aware of the matter, as none have seen its form."[59] Another of the authors added a few more details to the description, "It first is manifest in the countenance, but is not perceived by the body. . . . It has form but does not have form, and so no one is aware of the truth of matters."[60]

Like *Master Han Fei*, the *Inner Classic* was adamant that the healer, sometimes described as a sage, had to act early, *before* the patient began to feel discomfort. The "sagely healer moreover does not allow the illness to take shape," while the inferior craftsman only "watches that which is full-blown" or "intervenes when there has already been a defeat from an attack."[61] Such remarks were scattered throughout the text. "That which is invisible to the crude craftsman," the authors observed, "is precisely what the superior craftsman values."[62] The latter, the authors wrote, "guards the gates and windows" against illness. He moreover did not just rely upon the symptoms reported by patients, but instead acted prophylactically. He checked the pulse and watched the appearance for early signs or "sprouts" of illness.[63] The author drove home the idea through one analogy: "To use the poisons and medicines when the illness is already full-blown, to treat when the disturbance has taken shape – this is like digging a well when thirsty or casting weapons when war has broken out. Is it not too late?"[64]

Later medieval treatises on the curative arts go even further than the *Inner Classic*. They not only echoed the ideas found in *Master Han Fei* but also used the episode to illustrate the importance of preventive action. The *Training of the Heart from the Cinnabar Spring* (*Danxi xinfa* 丹溪心法) by the famous medical authority, Zhu Danxi 朱丹溪 (1281–1358), provides a final example. In this text, Zhu urged healers to "treat those who have yet to ail rather than those who already ail." For Zhu, patients who exhibited full-blown symptoms were lost causes, because the presence of overt symptoms indicated that the illness had already become critical. Bian Que's encounter with Lord Huan exemplified this principle. When Bian Que observed that the illness of Lord Huan had reached the inner recesses of the body, Zhu noted, "he determined that the lord could not be saved."[65]

The similarities between the metaphors of the Warring States persuaders and medical texts of the first century BC and beyond are striking. Just as earlier persuaders had creatively adapted elements of medical theory to craft a powerful message about the necessity of preventive action, later medical authors availed themselves of the imaginative potential of metaphors. In the process of reassembling textual fragments into literal pieces of history, such authors found new uses for old political allegories. And in this particular case, they discovered that the "ills that do not ail" not only made for catchy stories but were also "good to think with."[66]

3

CHUNYU YI: CAN THE HEALER SPEAK?

OUR DISCUSSION HAS REVEALED THE ROLE IN CREATING THE images of the medical fathers played by parties other than healers: the chroniclers who described the activities of a medical attendant from Qin, the persuaders who reshaped the image of the legendary Bian Que after the sagacious minister, and the historian who converted political allegories into biographical information. But what has yet to be seen in my story is the voice of the healer. How did healers represent themselves? Did they even represent themselves and if so, to what end?

In order to hear the healer's account of history, we require a change of scene. Following the unification of China in 221 BC, the kinds of stories told about healers began to change. This is not to say that the great healers of the Spring and Autumn (771–453 BC) failed to capture the imagination of writers. On the contrary, the distant past continued to exert its inexorable pull. New tales of Bian Que – tales that rivaled older fables in their dramatic flair – proliferated in the years following unification. At the same time, hints of a new interest in more contemporary and prosaic settings also appear. After the second century BC, there are glimpses of healers treating less exalted clients in small provincial "courts," conversing with colleagues in private drawing rooms, working in the makeshift infirmaries of the Central Asian frontier, trading herbs and more exotic substances in the marketplace, and even languishing in the jailhouses and dungeons of the imperial capital.

It is in this more contemporary setting that our next subject, another of Needham's medical fathers, Chunyu Yi (fl. ca. 180–154 BC), makes his first appearance in the historical record. Needham's discussion of Chunyu Yi points in no uncertain terms to the healer's biography in the *Records of the Grand Historian* of Sima Qian, which relates the healer's life in the following way.

Chunyu Yi had been arrested and transported to the capital in the west after being denounced for a serious crime (either around 176 or 167 BC, depending on the account).[1] According to Sima Qian, the accusation, left unspecified, was motivated by personal animosity: "Chunyu Yi had much success in determining whether the patient would live or die, but there were people whom he did not treat, and so their relatives bore a grudge against him." Confronted with the prospects of her father being severely punished or even executed, Chunyu's youngest daughter forwarded a memorial to the court, offering herself in his place. The memorial not only moved the emperor to spare the father but also to abolish all punishments involving the mutilation of the body. Sometime later, Chunyu Yi found himself dealing with the authorities once more, but this time answering to an imperial decree commanding him to describe his training and record of successful prognoses, a description now contained in the *Records of the Grand Historian*.[2]

According to modern historians, Chunyu Yi's biography in the *Records of the Grand Historian* provides a rare glimpse of how healers thought about medical practice and theory during the Han dynasty. To quote Lu and Needham, the records in the biography represent "the precious gift of a deep insight into the thoughts, the knowledge and the practice of a Chinese physician. . . ."[3] Even Elisabeth Hsu, the most skeptical reader of the *Records of the Grand Historian*, affirms its value as a source of medical history. In this connection, she writes, "The *Memoir* [i.e., the biography of the Granary Master] furthermore tells us about the transmission of medical knowledge and practice, names of a variety of 'medical' treatises and throws light on early developments in the history of Chinese therapeutics, in particular, of decoctions, acupuncture and moxibustion."[4]

Interestingly, early and medieval Chinese authors cast Chunyu Yi in a different light. In his origins narrative, Huangfu Mi compares Chunyu Yi to Attendant He. "Their analyses," Huangfu Mi observes, "captured root principles and thus they *did far more than just examine the ill*" (emphasis added).[5] The comparison is suggestive. As seen in Chapter 1, the description of Attendant He's efforts should be read less as a literal account of medical happenings than as a reflection on statecraft. This raises the question as to whether Huangfu Mi thought that the description of Chunyu Yi's activities also carried political resonance.

What is more, most of the earliest discussions of Chunyu Yi omit any and all reference to his career as a healer, focusing instead on his purported role in initiating penal – and thus political – reform during the Han.[6] No mentions of Chunyu's activities as a healer appear in the *Annals of Emperor Wen* (*Wendi benji* 文帝本紀) by Sima Qian or in a later chronicle, the *History of Han* (*Hanshu* 漢書), for example.[7] The famous memorial by Chunyu Yi's daughter, widely quoted and admired by early authors, similarly says nothing about her father's healing ability. In it, Chunyu Yi's daughter presents her father only as an official known for his "incorruptibility and impartiality."[8] The *Biography of Virtuous Women* (*Lienü zhuan* 列女傳), which dates to the late first century BC, also passes over Chunyu's track record of healing in silence. Instead, it chooses to identify Chunyu Yi as a granary official when relating how his daughter's bold plea moved the emperor to abolish mutilating punishments.[9] Given his political prominence, it need not surprise that early sources refer to Chunyu Yi not by name but by an official-sounding sobriquet, the "Granary Master," or "His Honor the Granary [Head]" (*Canggong* 倉公). Such a name invoked Chunyu Yi's position as the Head of the Great Granary of Qi, and it was used by virtually all ancient authors, including Sima Qian and Huangfu Mi.[10]

The stark differences between ancient and modern presentations of Chunyu Yi deserve explanation. Rather than trying to determine which is the more faithful, I investigate whether the two presentations of the figure, the healer and the official, can be reconciled. Should one think of the Chunyu Yi found in the *Records of the Grand Historian* as revealing an official face of medicine, and if so, who created this persona?

Before providing a road map of arguments to come, I offer the following clarification. As we shall see, a distinction should be made between the figure represented in a text of the first century BC and the actual personage of the second century BC.[11] For this reason, the former will be referred to as the "Granary Master," whereas the latter will be called "Chunyu Yi" throughout the chapter.

Caveats aside, this chapter uses the case of the Granary Master to investigate whether ancient healers had a hand in shaping the image of the medical fathers. After explaining my sources, I tackle the first part of this question: identifying the template for the persona in the *Records of the Grand Historian*. By examining the structure and logic of the descriptions of treatment in Sima Qian's biography, I show that the Granary Master is presented as reasoning and writing like a Han official. Having identified the archetype for the Granary Master's persona, I then turn to question who it was that created this official face of medicine. While it is uncertain whether the descriptions of treatment were actually written by the historical Chunyu Yi; Sima Qian did *not* fabricate the document or the figure of the Granary Master *ex novo* either. Most likely, the historian drew upon materials produced by imperial officials, officials who had documented their efforts to heal in a manner reminiscent of the Granary Master. As the final analysis shall reveal, such officials, however, did not write about healing out of an inherent interest in the subject; rather, they detailed their efforts to cure as an extension of their administrative duties.

SETTING THE STAGE

The last chapter ended just as the Qin state was poised to conquer all of China. By the time the Granary Master had reached maturity, however, the Qin empire had already come and gone. Although the achievements of the Qin were undeniable – they created an impressive legal apparatus, a comprehensive transportation and communication infrastructure, and an innovative administrative strategy of ruling through imperial proxies – the dynasty did not last more than a generation before a modest uprising brought it to a swift end in 206 BC. The uprising was followed by a civil war; bandits and local magnates seized the opportunity to reassert their power, and the scions of the aristocratic houses conquered by the Qin resurfaced, eager to reclaim their patrimony.

It was in this context that Liu Bang 劉邦 (r. 206–195 BC), a man of obscure origin, founded the Han dynasty. When he claimed the Qin title of emperor after the civil war, Liu Bang did not have the power to return to the centralized arrangement of the Qin. Under these circumstances, it is unsurprising that Liu Bang agreed to an arrangement in which the "empire" comprised a large number of semiautonomous kingdoms, many of which were in the east. One of these was the home state of Chunyu Yi (see Figure 8). As one might expect, many of the rulers of these kingdoms fancied themselves the equals of the Han emperor and entertained dynastic ambitions of their own. Faced with such bald challenges to their authority as well as open rebellions, Liu Bang's successors, including the emperor who would pardon Chunyu Yi, required little persuasion to reassert control. By the time that Sima Qian wrote his biography, the era of the kings was over. The emperors had broken their power, abolishing the kingdoms in which Chunyu Yi had purportedly lived and practiced his curative skills (see Figure 9).

With the context thus explained, we turn to sources. This chapter will focus on the portions of the *Records of the Grand Historian* relating to Chunyu Yi, or the second half of the "Biographies of Bian Que and the

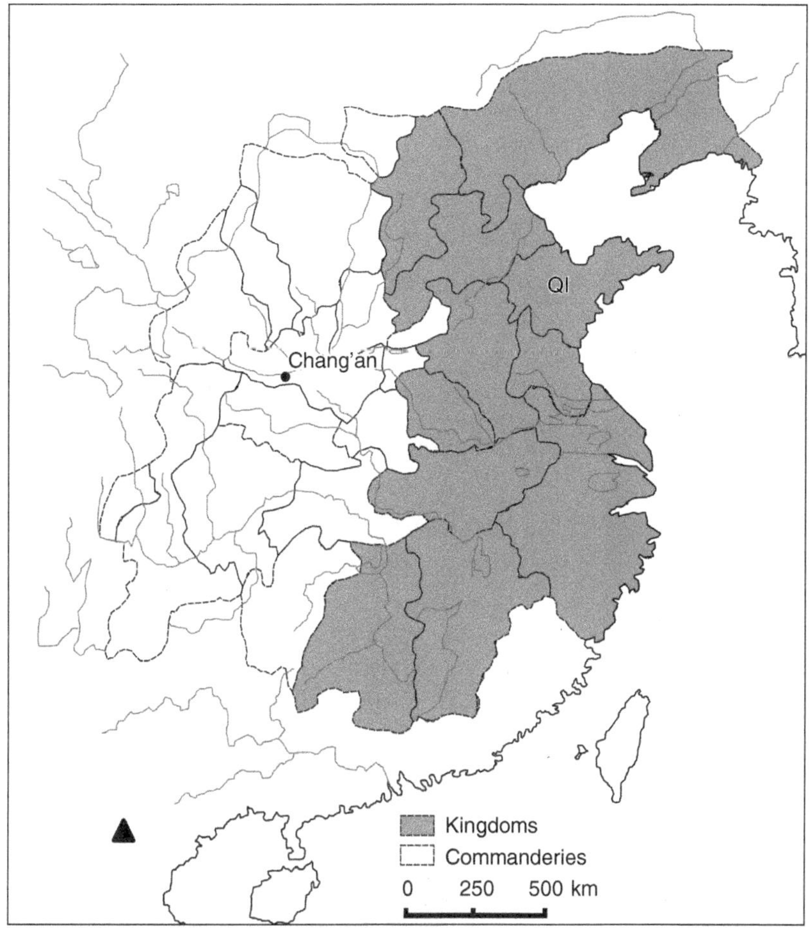

Figure 8 Map of the Han empire and the feudatories, ca. 195 BC. The Granary Master, the subject of this chapter, hailed from the eastern feudatory of Qi.

Source: Drawn by Daniel Shultz after map in *Cambridge History of China: Volume 1: The Ch'in and Han Empires, 221 B.C.–A.D. 220*, edited by Denis Twitchett and Michael Loewe (1986), 125. Adapted with permission from Cambridge University Press.

Granary Master." The larger organization of this half, which is complex and intricate, is represented schematically in Figure 10. It opens with a capsule sketch of the Granary Master: his origins, training, and questions from the authorities regarding his medical activities.[12] The narrative then moves briskly to what appears to have been the Granary Master's lengthy response to queries from the authorities, some of which repeats (and contradicts) information already set forth in the capsule sketch. This

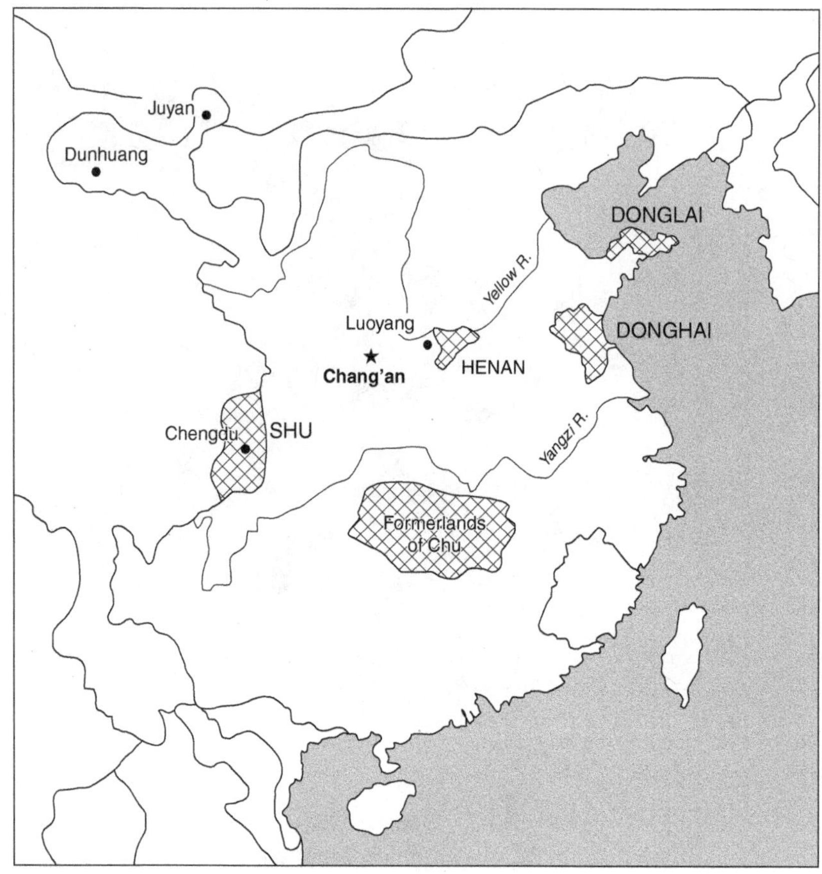

Figure 9 Map of Han empire in 108 BC. The political landscape of China in Sima Qian's day offers a sharp contrast to that of the Granary Master.

Source: Michael Loewe, *Bing: From Farmer's Son to Magistrate in Han China* (2011). Reproduced with permission from Hackett Publishing Company, all rights reserved.

document, which I refer to as the Granary Master's response, can be further divided into three parts: (1) a description of the Granary Master's training;[13] (2) twenty-five descriptions of encounters with the ill, or the records of consultation (henceforth, the Granary Master's records);[14] (3) and eight answers to official queries.[15] The biography then closes with Sima Qian's final remarks, where the histories of Bian Que and the Granary Master are compared.[16]

Besides the biography of the Granary Master, this chapter considers other early texts with comparable formats. These include the logs

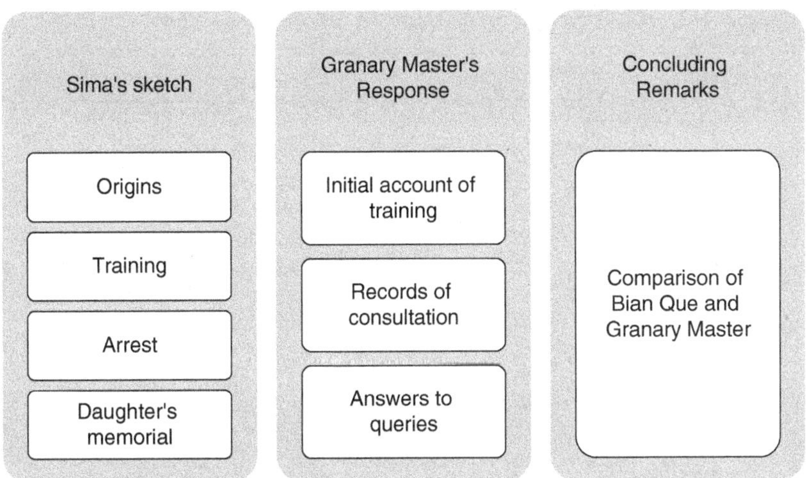

Figure 10 Sima Qian's biography of the Granary Master. The organization of the chapter is complex, and the historian drew from a range of heterogeneous sources.
Source: Image drawn by author.

of divination recovered by archaeologists from tombs, dating to the fourth century BC, discussed briefly in the first chapter. As we shall see, many of these logs relate the results of medical divinations performed on behalf of a sick nobleman. Additionally, our discussion encompasses the administrative documents unearthed near former Qin and Han dynasty military settlements and administrative offices, as well as the tombs of local officials in Northwest and South Central China.[17] (For a list of sites, see Table 4.) The contents of these documents vary, and included material as miscellaneous as household registers, grain and weapons inventories, official communications, ordinances, statutes, model memoranda, and a collection of twenty-two legal case summaries (*zouyan shu* 奏讞書). The case summaries, discussed at length in the following text, deserve explanation. Dating between the late third and early second centuries BC, such summaries report instances in which reaching a decision proved difficult, and so local officials petitioned the Ministry of Justice for a decision. Judging from a Qin dynasty manuscript with similar contents bought from the Hong Kong antiquities market, the summaries belonged to a broader genre of pedagogical texts that circulated in early official circles.[18] The readership of such summaries was most likely local officials who sometimes bore the responsibility of deciding legal cases.[19]

Table 4 *Sites with Administrative Documents Discussed in This Chapter*

	Site Name	Date	Location	Type of Site
1	Shuihudi 睡虎地	Ca. 217 BC	Yunmeng, Hubei (SC China)	Tomb
2	Liye 里耶	Qin dynasty	Hunan (SC China)	Trash deposits
3	Yuelu 岳麓	Qin dynasty	Unknown	Unknown
4	Zhangjiashan 張家山	Ca. 186 BC	Hubei (SW China)	Tomb
5	Lianyungang 連雲港	Ca. 50 BC–AD 8	Jiangsu (SW China)	Tomb
6	Juyan 居延	Ca. 110 BC–AD 95	Gansu (NW China)	
7	Dunhuang 敦煌	Ca. 98 BC–AD 137	Gansu (NW China)	
8	Yinwan 尹灣	10 BC	Jiangsu (SE China)	Tomb
9	Wuwei Hantanpo 武威旱灘坡	Early first century AD	Gansu (NW China)	Tomb

As we shall see, the formats of the legal summaries and other kinds of bureaucratic documents were distinct from other forms of writing in early China. We can thus use the format and styles of reasoning to determine who fashioned the persona of the Granary Master.

THE HEALER AS AN OFFICIAL?

While it may seem like a foregone conclusion that the Granary Master's response would only present the figure as a healer, there are reasons to suspect otherwise. The language of Sima Qian's biography leaves the impression that the diagnosis and treatment of ills was akin to legal decision making, the latter being one of the responsibilities of early officials. The Granary Master, for example, referred to the act of issuing a prognosis as the judgment (*jue* 決) or decision (*duan* 斷), two terms also used for the sentences handed down by early officials. He furthermore called the checking of the pulse and appearance the examinations (*zhen* 診), a move that highlighted the similarities between crime and illness. The Granary Master, finally, spoke of the tools for differentiating between types of illnesses as *fa* (法), a turn of phrase that recalls the official's practice of

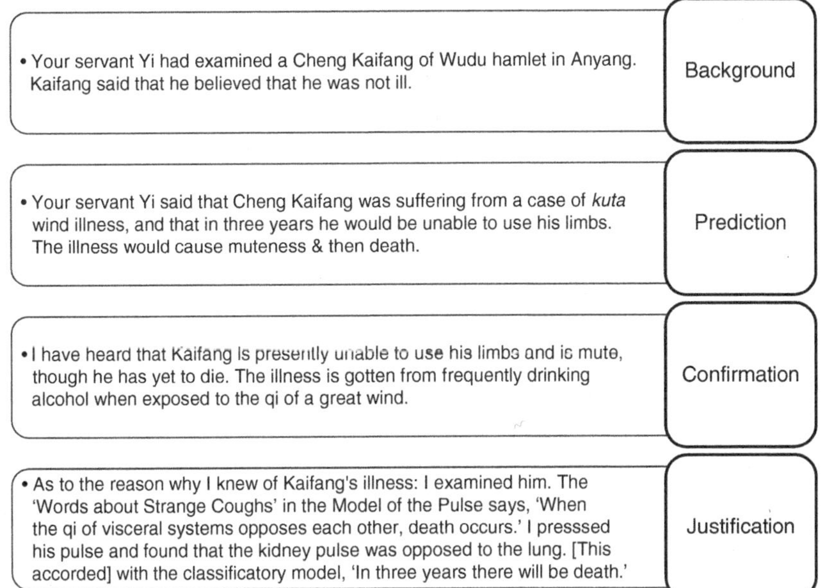

Figure 11 The Granary Master's record at a glance. One of the Granary Master's twenty-five records of consultation preserved in the *Records of the Grand Historian* (ca. 90 BC).

Source: Image drawn by author.

"using the legal classes to adjudicate an offense (*yi fa lun* 以法論)."[20] Though intriguing, the implications of such legal resonances have yet to be pursued by historians.[21] In this section, I thus compare the records of consultation to contemporary legal documents, showing that the format of the Granary Master's records mirrors the logic and structure of the legal case summaries. Such resemblances, it will be furthermore demonstrated, indicate that the Granary Master was presented in the records of consultation as an official.

In this connection, it would be instructive to examine one of the Granary Master's records in detail, which has been translated and analyzed in Figure 11.[22] As the figure reveals, the structure falls into four parts: the background, prognosis, confirmation, and justification. The background relates the essential information of the case: his or her place of registration, name, status, as well as the circumstances behind the healer's encounter with the sick person. The prognosis sets forth the Granary Master's initial assessment of the illness, including his determination of the agent of the sickness. The confirmation, in turn, records the actual outcome of the illness: for example, when the patient died or the method of treatment, and the time of resolution. The justification, finally, reveals the process by which the Granary Master purportedly arrived at his prognosis. Generally, this justification is marked off with a single phrase, "The way that I learned of the illness of so-and-so" (*suoyi zhi . . . bingzhe* 所以知...病者). Before we turn to other texts with analogous formats, it is worth emphasizing that Figure 11 is representative of the structure of most of the Granary Master's records. As Elisabeth Hsu demonstrates, such records were highly formulaic and thus varied little in their structure.[23]

A similar, though not identical, format appears in many of the surviving legal case summaries excavated from the Zhangjiashan tomb (ca. 186 BC), which contain materials dating close to the time of Chunyu Yi. The majority of the summaries may be analyzed into four different parts. The first sets forth the *background* information, in which the author fills in the information about the crime in question: the malefactor's place of registration and official rank or position, as well as the salient facts of the case. The second or *judgment* includes the official's decision regarding the proper category to which the crime was to be assigned and the corresponding sentence. In this respect, it resembled the Granary Master's prognosis, which depended on properly categorizing the illness. The third part was the official's *justification* for assigning a crime to a particular legal category, a subject to which we will return. Finally, the fourth might be thought of as a *confirmation*: here, the officials from the Ministry of Justice would either confirm or overturn the decision of local officials regarding the nature of the offense.[24] The legal summaries are less consistent than the Granary Master's records in their format. The sequence of the four parts of the case summaries – when they were presented in full – actually varied. In most cases, the judgment followed the justification, but in others, the sequence was closer to that found in the Granary Master's records, as the justification preceded the confirmation.

The inclusion of justifications in both the Granary Master's records and the earlier legal case summaries is telling. This is because the justification, often the longest part of the Granary Master's records, was uncommon in early Chinese documents. It is in the justification that the Granary Master recounted the process by which he arrived at his prognosis. In the case of Cheng Kaifang 成開方, mentioned in Figure 11, the Granary Master's prediction about the man's imminent death was based on the fact that the pulse from the kidney system was opposed to that of the lung, an observation that fit with the pattern of "the *qi* from the visceral systems being opposed to each other." His prognosis of the man's time of death was also drawn from the same text, which noted that death would occur within the next three years.

The case of Cheng Kaifang is hardly unique. Most of the justifications in the Granary Master's records follow a common pattern of explaining his observations in relation to authoritative texts. Another record relates the case of a man who died from an illness gotten from engaging in sexual intercourse while in a rage. In this connection, the Granary Master noted: "I stopped his pulse and got a hot reading from the lungs." And to explain how such a reading led him to infer imminent death, the Granary Master juxtaposed a description of the man's pulse with the following passage from a lost text, the *Model of the Pulse* (*Maifa* 脈法)[25]: "If the pulse is uneven but drumlike, the body will dissipate." When the Granary Master examined the man, he noticed a very similar pattern. The pulse, he wrote, was "uneven at times and intermittent." Although the man's pulse was not identical to the textual description, the Granary Master nevertheless realized that it was analogous enough and so inferred that the man was suffering from an illness that caused the dissipation of the body.[26] The examples cited in the preceding text are typical of the justifications. Very few of them, in fact, diverge from the pattern of juxtaposing the healer's observation of the appearance and pulse against passages drawn from an authoritative work.

Justifications, it should be emphasized, were quite uncommon in early Chinese texts. Take the case of the divinatory logs dating to the fourth century BC. Like the Granary Master's records, these logs are highly formulaic in their structure, something pointed out by the modern scholar Li Ling 李零.[27] The logs also share a common format with the records of the Granary Master, all arriving at an illation through a three-pronged defense containing background information, a prediction, and finally, a confirmation (see Figure 12).[28] Similarities notwithstanding, there is one difference worth marking: the justifications are absent from extant divinatory logs from the Warring States. Such logs are silent as to how diviners arrived at their judgments as to the agent and outcome of illness. What signs in the tortoise shells and milfoil stalks caused them to imagine that the sick man or woman would recover? And how did they arrive at the identity of the agent, or make a determination about the proper sacrificial solution? If later manuals, which set forth diagrams for

• In the year [after] Grand Minister of War Dao Gu led the Chu forces to rescue Fu, on the month of *xinyi* (first month?), *jimao* day (sixteenth day in the sexagenary calendar), Gu Ji used the *baojia* [methods] to divine on behalf of Minister on the Left [Shao] Tuo: [He has] already been afflicted with an illness of the abdomen and heart (belly?), and because of the rising *qi*, he cannot relish his food, and the illness has lingered for a long time without being cured. May he be quickly cured and there be no baleful influence.	Background
• The divination is entirely auspicious, although the illness will be difficult to cure. According to its agents, make *shuo* sacrifices. Make a pledge sacrifice to the Great Unity of the [sacrificial] meat of one [young (tender)] lamb or sheep; to the Lord of Earth and the Director of Life each of one ewe. Make a pledge sacrifice of the [sacrificial] meat of one young ox to the Great Waters; to the Two Sons of Heaven each of one ewe; to Mount Gui, one black whole ram. Make a pledge sacrifice of two black whole rams to Chu ancestors Laotong, Zhu Rong (The Lord of Fire?), and Yuxiong, offering an Enjoyment Sacrifice to them. Make a Steam Sacrifice to the High and Low Hills, each of one whole pig. May Shao Tuo return to his original state [of health]. We will make an attacking and repelling exorcism of the Jupiter year star.	Prediction
• Gu Ji prognosticated it and said: Auspicious.	Confirmation

Figure 12 A divinatory record from the Baoshan site (late fourth century BC). Like the Granary Master's records, the background of divinatory records relates the name of the patient, the ailments that occasioned a divination, and the methods used by the diviner to determine the agent and sacrificial solution to illness.

Source: Image drawn by author.

reading tortoise shells or interpreting dreams are any indication of earlier practices, these Warring States diviners had a system for interpreting the cracks or stalks.[29] Yet for whatever reason, they did not feel the need to justify their reasoning – at least in writing.

Indeed, the justification was so uncommon that it is missing from other surviving representations of medical reasoning. The closest analogue to the justification is found in the story of the Prince of Guo 虢, recounted in the biography of Bian Que.[30] Before delving into the details of our analysis, it might be useful to rehearse the rough outlines of the case. The prince had suddenly fallen into a deathlike state, leading everyone in the palace to believe that he had died. Before the body could be shrouded for burial, Bian Que arrived at the gates of the palace, only to be met by the grieving brother of the Crown Prince. Much to the mourner's surprise, Bian Que, *without* examining the patient, announced that the Crown Prince had *not* died but was just unconscious. The famed healer then proposed to treat the Crown Prince and, with several disciples, set to reviving the sick man.[31]

Bearing the foregoing outline in mind, we can proceed to explain the differences between the tale of Bian Que and the Granary Master's records. Some elements in Bian Que's story do come close to a justification (but not quite). In delivering his prognosis, Bian Que related the progress of the illness: the chain of events that began with a disturbance in the viscera and culminated in the prince's falling into a deathlike slumber. And insofar as it too exhibits a high degree of technical detail, the description of the progress of the illness resembles the Granary Master's records. Yet for all their apparent similarities, Bian Que's etiology lacks an account of how the mythical healer arrived at his prognosis. Instead, Bian Que behaved like a magician or wonderworker. In this story, he is said to have announced that the "dead" prince was actually alive while standing *outside* of the gates of the palace – that is, prior to laying eyes upon the patient. Needless to say, Bian Que's reasoning represents something of a black box: Was Bian Que able to "see" the patient from the other side of the gates with his penetrating vision, or were the secondhand reports about the prince sufficient? And what texts or tools did Bian Que use as the basis for his inferences? Bian Que said nothing, and so we will never know. The mysterious, or better still, the miraculous, nature of Bian Que's prognosis is underscored by his challenge to a skeptical interlocutor, a challenge familiar to fans of magic shows. "If you sir take my words as being devoid of truth," Bian Que told the brother of the "dead" prince, "then enter the private chambers and examine the Crown Prince; you should be able to hear ringing from his ears and the swelling of his nostrils, and if you rub the area from his two thighs reaching down to his privates," Bian Que added, "you will find it still to be warm."[32]

Instead, the legal case summaries of Han are the only surviving documents with the kind of justification found in the Granary Master's records. Dating to the second century BC, these summaries supply the earliest surviving effort to explicate the facts of the case and anchor them to the statutes. Consider one of the cases involving a county magistrate who had conspired with his subordinates to murder a former colleague. After the murder, the magistrate had his henchmen apprehended before secretly ordering them to be released in a fake jailbreak to cover up his role in the whole sordid affair. When officials from above came to investigate the disappearance, they discovered the plot and promptly condemned the guilty parties to death. They justified the sentences in the following way:

Observation	鞫(鞫)之: 蒼賊殺人, 信與謀。丙, 贅捕蒼而縱之。審。敢言之。新鄭信, 髳長蒼謀賊殺獄史武, 校長丙, 贅捕蒼而縱之。爵皆大庶長。	We did an interrogation by beating: Cang had murdered someone, after having plotted together with Xin. Bing and Zhui had arrested Cang but released him. This has all been borne out by investigation. We dare to say that Xin of Xinqi and Cang, head of Mao, plotted to murder the prison scribe, Wu. The bureau head, Bing, together with Zhui captured Cang and released him. Their ranks within the [twenty] orders of honor were eighteenth.
Authoritative Text	律: 賊殺人, 棄市。	According to the statutes: those who murder someone are to be executed with the corpses discarded in the marketplace.
Inference	以此當蒼。	It is on this basis that we determined Cang's punishment.
Authoritative Text	律: 謀賊殺人, 與賊同法。	The statutes also observe: "To plot to murder falls under the same class as the criminal offense of robbing or killing them."
Inference	以此當信。	It is on this basis that we have made a determination about Xin's punishment.
Authoritative Text	律: 縱囚, 與同罪。	According to the statutes: "He who releases a prisoner will share the same punishment as the prisoner."
Inference	以此當丙, 贅, 當之, 信, 蒼, 丙, 贅皆當棄市, 毄 (繫) 。	It is on this basis that we have made a determination about Bing and Zhui. We have determined as follows: Xin, Cang, Bing, and Zhui are to be executed and their corpses discarded in the marketplace. They are to be bound immediately for the sentence.[33]

The structure of the justification in the legal case summaries resembles those found in the Granary Master's records. The progression from an investigation of the facts of the case to a final judgment parallels the Granary Master's move from the "examination" of bodily signs to the prognosis. Just as the Granary Master described all of the salient features of an illness, officials noted the relevant testimonies and methods of interrogation – for example, whether torture was used. More importantly, the issuing of a sentence in the legal case summaries is akin to the route by which the Granary Master arrived at a prognosis. Once the facts could be established in a judicial case, the officials justified their classification of the offense by interlacing descriptions of the case's particulars with citations from the statutes. Such a move, in fact, mirrors the Granary Master's explanations of his own prognoses; he too juxtaposed the reading of the pulse with passages from authoritative texts. Moreover, in explaining how they decided upon a sentence, the officials would also cite the relevant statutes that applied. Such a move resonated with the Granary Master's habit of explicating his prognosis by citing a passage from an authoritative work like the *Model of the Pulse.*

A comparison of the Granary Master's records of consultation and earlier legal case summaries thus discloses striking structural and logical parallels between the two. The parallels are all the more revealing when one considers that the elements found in both sets of documents were relatively uncommon, increasing the likelihood that the Granary Master's records were patterned directly after the legal case summaries. In other words, the impression left by the official name of the Granary Master is more than coincidental. The persona in the *Records of the Grand Historian* wrote like an official.

WHOSE VOICE?

We have shown thus far that in the *Records of the Grand Historian,* the Granary Master was presented as reasoning and documenting his efforts to cure like an official, but this still does not tell us who created this persona. To answer this question, I take a second look at the Granary Master's response. As we shall see, the murky provenance of Sima Qian's sources frustrates efforts to establish whether the historical figure wrote the text. At the same time, it is unlikely that Sima Qian conjured the Granary Master's official persona from thin air. By comparing the contents of the Granary Master's response, and in particular the records of consultation, I argue that Sima Qian drew upon material left behind by someone like the historical Chunyu Yi, probably an official familiar with administrative practices of documenting efforts to track and to treat sickness.

Before explaining the reasons to the contrary, I begin with the received view, because scholars have long regarded the Granary Master's response as the work of the historical Chunyu Yi. Christopher Cullen, for example, argues that the description sets forth a "transcription of the text of the annotated interrogatory from official files," a position also held by other scholars.[34] Admittedly, the received view is rather inviting. To begin with, it is consistent with the fact that the response in the biography is narrated in the first person. Throughout the response, the author refers to himself as "Your servant Yi" (*chen Yi* 臣意), which suggests that he is none other than Chunyu Yi. In addition, the response seems to have been reproduced from a single document, because Sima Qian does not, at any point, interrupt the narrative presented in the Granary Master's voice.

There is another virtue to the received view. If the official format and tone of the Granary Master's records belonged to the hand of the historical Chunyu Yi, then they could easily be explained. As mentioned previously, Chunyu Yi had been the head of the royal granaries in his home state. As a local official, he would thus have been familiar with the conventions of drafting official memoranda. He would also have known how to present his medical reasoning in a manner readily accessible to other members of the bureaucracy. Indeed, one might even suspect that when faced with inquiries from court about his activities as a healer, Chunyu Yi would have found it expedient to fall back on bureaucratic ways of thinking and organizing information.

For all of its appeal, the received view has been challenged by Michael Loewe, Jin Shiqi, and Elisabeth Hsu. They question whether the Granary Master's response was actually as it appears: a single document submitted to the court at the time of Chunyu Yi's incarceration. Both Michael Loewe and Jin Shiqi note that the Granary Master's response contains anachronistic references and internal inconsistencies that undermine the appearance of unity. Crucially, the Granary Master mentioned that his teacher had been dead for a decade, a comment that could not have been made after 167 BC due to internal evidence.[35] Yet a number of the Granary Master's records discussed events that postdate his arrest by decades: for example, a rebellion of princes in 154 BC. Although these do not rule out Chunyu Yi's authorship of the Granary Master's response for either Loewe or Jin Shiqi, the discrepancies nevertheless suggest that Sima Qian had merged materials composed at different times into a single document.[36]

Additionally, Chunyu Yi's authorship of the Granary Master's response has been challenged by Elisabeth Hsu. Pointing to "incongruencies in medical rationale and terminology," Hsu argues that there are editorial interventions and insertions in the response that postdate the lifetime of Chunyu Yi. According to her, the first ten cases of the Granary Master's records can be seen as a mirror of medical knowledge in Chunyu Yi's day, that is, between 180 and 177 BC. The rest of the response, she notes, should be regarded as later additions "based on stories reflecting later but related medical understandings from a variety of localities and time periods." Hsu continues, explaining that Sima Qian "may have edited these texts in his own prose, which reflects early first-century currents of medical knowledge." Like so many other early Chinese texts, the biography of the Granary Master was heterogeneous in origin. Some of the contents, she writes, were by the hand of the historical Chunyu Yi, whereas others were not.[37]

The arguments advanced by Loewe and others undermine the received view on the authorship of the Granary Master's response, but can we find evidence of any healer's voice within Sima Qian's biography? There are reasons to wonder. If, as we saw in Chapter 2, Sima Qian intended the histories of the Granary Master and Bian Que to serve as metaphors for the dangers facing officials, then it would make sense that he would edit documents to look like legal summaries. By calling attention to the parallels between the Granary Master and the official, Sima Qian would be able to enhance the rhetorical effect of the biography.

Although the editorial license exercised by Sima Qian should not be discounted, it is nevertheless unlikely that the historian created the Granary Master's persona from nothing. In point of fact, Sima Qian generally recycled and rearranged existing material, a habit that won him the reputation as a "scissors-and-paste" historian.[38] Additionally, as Loewe points out, the language of the Granary Master stands in relief to the rest of the chapter, which is written with Sima Qian's usual polish. Such a discrepancy points to the fact that Sima Qian had refrained from editing his sources, and so the response is best thought of as a "raw copy."[39] Because of this, Loewe concludes that the biography contains a "greater proportion of primary material" than most of the other chapters in the *Records of the Grand Historian.* The inconsistencies within the chapter furthermore support Loewe's assertion that Sima Qian edited materials lightly. The surname of the Granary Master's teacher is rendered differently throughout the chapter. More strikingly, the biography includes contradictory accounts of the Granary Master's training. In his introductory remarks, Sima Qian claims that Chunyu's master was Yang Qing 陽慶, a man without children: "Yang Qing was over seventy and had no children; he asked Chunyu Yi to discard all of his old formulas and bestowed on him Yang's secret formulas." In the second version, in which the Granary Master responded to various queries, the biography states that Yang did in fact have children. One of them purportedly had been a friend of Chunyu Yi, and even introduced the future court physician to the father.[40]

Our foregoing discussion raises the question as to where Sima Qian got the raw materials – particularly the descriptions of diagnosis and treatment – from which to create the Granary Master's response. As the Grand Scribe of the Han, we would expect Sima Qian to have had a wide array of sources in the imperial archives at his disposal, including copies and summaries of administrative documents.[41] This is no trivial point. The balance of this chapter will show that administrative documents resemble the Granary Master's records so much in terms of content that the author of the latter was probably someone like the historical Chunyu Yi, that is, a local official familiar with keeping sick logs and medical records.

So what evidence is there to suggest that an official would have written the Granary Master's records – or, at least, furnished the raw materials that Sima Qian later rearranged? While modern historians may treat the healing arts and state governance as distinct disciplines, in Sima Qian's time, the realms of the medic and magistrate were quite miscible. This is revealed by the sheer number of formulas copied by officials recovered from early imperial sites. Consider the following excerpts, taken from manuscripts dating to the Qin and Han dynasties respectively:

> 病暴心痛灼灼者, 治之, 析蓂實, 冶二; 枯橿(薑), 菌桂, 冶 各一。凡三物并和, 取三指最 (撮) 到節二, 溫醇酒。
>
> To treat those stricken with a violent eruption of heart pain that burns: Pulverize two seeds of Pennycress. Pulverize one dried ginger and one Cassia twig. Combine all three of these substances. Take a three-finger pinch, knuckle deep, warming it with concentrated wine....[42]
>
> 治久欬逆[43]。 匈 (胸) 庳 (痹)。 痿 庳 (痹) 。 止泄心腹。 久積, 傷寒方。 人參, 茈宛 (紫菀) , 昌蒲, 細辛, 薑, 桂, 蜀椒各一分。烏喙十分。皆合和。 以
>
> [...] to treat those suffering from persistent coughs and reversal, numbness in the heart, and atrophy [in the extremities]; to stop leakage

> from the heart and abdomen (i.e., diarrhea or loose bowels), persistent accumulations in the heart and abdomen: a formula for cold damage disorders.
>
> One *fen* (3 g) each of ginseng, Purple Aster, Sweetflag or Calamus, Chinese wild ginger, ginger, Cassia twigs, Szechun pepper; and 10 *fen* (35 g) of monkshood root. Combine all of these. With....[44]

Worth noting here is the location where the formulas were found. They were discovered *not* in the personal or family tombs of officials but rather in the discarded archives of administrative offices. Similar formulas have moreover been unearthed from sites throughout the empire: in the northwest frontier and in the south central heartland.[45] What is more, such formulas were located alongside a host of other administrative documents: personnel records, official depositions and correspondence, requests for leave, ledgers of accounts and transactions, passports, handwriting samples, official decrees, and legal statutes. This fact suggests that officials read about and experimented with formulas not only in their personal lives but also, more crucially, in an official capacity.

The role of dynastic representatives in administering health care on a routine basis makes it even more likely that the men furnishing the raw materials for the Granary Master's records, like the historical Chunyu Yi, had served as officials. Surviving administrative documents reveal that officials were involved in providing health care to members of their ranks as well as garrison forces. From at least Qin times, officials were charged with documenting the outbreak of epidemics. One manuscript indicates that authorities called upon healers to examine suspected victims of contagious illnesses and to record the dates of their examinations.[46] When not tracking epidemics, members of the bureaucracy also oversaw the treatment of illness, took responsibility for the transport and distribution of medicine, and supervised the application of acupuncture or moxa to those affected by plagues.[47] The interest in medical matters was more than humanitarian, as the health of dynastic subjects naturally had ramifications for imperial revenues and for the success of public works projects, campaigns, and military colonies.

There is another reason to suspect the officials of having supplied the raw materials for the Granary Master's records, specifically, the shared content between the Granary Master's records and the administrative documents. Early officials anticipated the Granary Master's habit of keeping records of consultation, or what the latter referred to as "charting out the records of examination, prognostications, and determinations about whether the patient would survive, and observing instances of success or failure."[48] Consider the following fragments:

> 田卒平干國襄垣石安里李彊, 年卅七, 本始五年二月丁未, 疾心腹丈(脹)滿, 死。右農前丞報。
>
> Li Qiang, a garrison soldier from Shi'an hamlet in Xiangyuan county of Pinggan Kingdom, aged thirty seven: On the forty-fourth day of the sexagenary cycle of the fifth year of the era of Original Beginnings (69 BC), Li became ill from distension in his heart and abdomen. He has died. The Front Assistant to the Agricultural Office of the Right reports.[49]

Another log, dating almost a century later (ca. 27 AD), similarly reads:

> 廼二月壬午病。加兩脾 (髀)雍 (癰) 種 (腫) 。匈 (胸) 脅丈(脹)滿。不耐食飲。未能視事。
>
> In the second month and the nineteenth day of the sexagenary cycle, I took ill. On top of this, I developed abscesses in both thighs and swelling in my upper chest area. I can no longer bear to eat or drink. I am not yet able to assume my duties.[50]

Though organized differently from the Granary Master's records, the sick logs kept by officials were very similar in terms of content. Like the Granary Master, the author included information about the sick person, his place of registration and official rank. In addition, the official's log was characterized by a lack of literary flourish – in particular, the parallel construction that distinguished stylists from less masterful writers. The vocabulary of illness also presented an element of commonality; as with the Granary Master's records, sick logs abounded with references to distended bellies and fullness (*zhangman* 脹滿), abscesses (*yong* 癰), swellings (*zhong* 腫), hot spells and chills, headaches, and so forth. Finally, and perhaps most strikingly, the official records revealed the same interest in temporal progression. Although the sick logs apparently did not contain prognostications, they recorded, much like the Granary Master's records of consultation, the initial onset of the illness, as well as the time to recovery or death.[51]

Besides recording incidences of illness, Qin and Han officials kept track of the successes and failures of treatment in a manner reminiscent of the Granary Master. In writing reports of treatment, these officials included the sick person's period of incapacitation, the chief symptoms, the nature and dosage of the treatment, results of treatment, and time to recovery.

One excerpt, taken from a score of administrative records, noted that a soldier had "a headache on the eighth day of the fourth month. He suffers from cold and hot spells, and drank five doses of medicine but has yet to improve."[52] Another log documented an effort to treat a soldier who had fallen ill. The log told not only that the man received moxibustion in two places as well as drugs to take, but also the name of the person who applied the treatment. Though incomplete, the log revealed that the same soldier was then treated by a healer and given two doses of medicine.[53] In this respect, the sick log recalls the Granary Master's penchant for keeping track of the previous, unsuccessful efforts of other healers. Perhaps the most striking of these records involved the treatment of a horse. Like the Granary Master's records, this one briefly described the salient features of the illness, the source of the drug formulas, and the number of days before the horse saw improvement and a full recovery.[54]

Who created the persona of the Granary Master in the *Records of the Grand Historian*? Although a definitive answer is elusive at this time, it seems unlikely that Sima Qian created the Granary Master single-handedly. Instead, the preponderance of evidence indicates that the historian fashioned the image of the figure by cobbling together existing textual resources. Such resources probably included the sick logs and records of consultation kept by officials, which resembled the Granary Master's records in terms of their contents. It thus seems fair to say that Han officials contributed the raw materials that Sima Qian would later use to make the persona in the *Records of the Grand Historian*.

FROM OFFICIAL MEMORANDUM TO CASE HISTORIES

As my discussion shows, determining whether healers spoke through the mouthpiece of the Granary Master is not as straightforward as it might seem. Such a question belies the fact that the Granary Master was a product of multiple hands. These include the historian and editor, Sima Qian, who told the story of the men who healed to expose the dangers of public life, as well as the early officials who practiced the curative arts as an extension of their administrative duties. For such officials, healing did not represent some kind of calling, occupation, or even subject of independent inquiry. For them, the curative arts were part of the business of governance, one of a host of duties pursued in the course of governing the realm: the surveying of frontiers, supervising of corvée laborers, conducting of criminal investigations, repairing of irrigation systems, and the building of walls. To put it differently, when such men wrote about sickness they did not do so as career *healers* but rather as imperial officials.

Sources composed after Sima Qian's time furthermore indicate that the official who healed was something of a stock figure to the early imperial elite. Consider one of a number of stories about the healing powers of Deng Xun 鄧訓 (36–92), who, like the Granary Master, had a formidable daughter (Deng's daughter would subsequently become the empress dowager and virtual ruler of China for decades). While serving in the northwest frontier, Deng's men were incapacitated by an epidemic, which spread like wildfire. In response, Deng Xun chose to handle the crisis personally. As his biographer explained: "He boiled the decoctions and medicines himself, and so all of the ill were cured."[55] A similar account also survives for an architect of the Imperial Palace who lived in the first century AD. According to his biographer, an epidemic had struck the laborers who were working on a project overseen by the official. The situation roused the architect to action. "He made rounds of inspection and went to the sick corvée laborers," the biographer noted, "personally seeing to the preparation of the medicines and porridge for the sick." Such efforts bore fruit, as "the number of men who died from illness was reduced."[56]

Indeed, the curative powers of officials were so well-known to early Chinese readers that they represented a selling point for formulas. Consider the following excerpt from a manuscript dating to the early first century AD. It relates a cure for unpleasant afflictions that plague the nether regions of men:

> 活樓根十分,天雄五分,牛膝四分,續斷四分,[...][...]五分,昌蒲二分,凡六物,皆并冶合,和以方寸匕一為後飯,㥁(愈)久病者。卅日平復,百日毋疾苦。建威耿將軍方,良,禁千金不傳也。
>
> 10 *fen* [35 g][57] of Trichosanthes roots; 5 *fen* [17 g] of aconite; 4 *fen* [14 g] of Achyranthes; 4 *fen* [14 g] of Szechuan teasel; 5 *fen* [17 g] of [lacunae]; 2 *fen* [7 g] of Sweetflag or Calamus.
>
> Pulverize and mix all six substances, combining and taking a square-inch spoonful after eating. The medicine will cure even those who have been long ill. In thirty days they will improve; in one hundred days, they will be without pain. A formula of General Geng of Jianwei. Excellent. Forbidden to transmit even for a thousand coins.[58]

What draws the eye here are two details, the first being the use of an official title in a medical text. Apparently, the Granary Master was not the only practitioner of the curative arts known by an official-sounding name. In addition, the reference to *General* Geng is also striking for several reasons. The Geng in question here has been identified by scholars as Geng Yan 耿弇 (3–58 AD), a high-ranking official, war hero, and member of a powerful ministerial clan.[59] Though it should not be accepted at face value, the ascription discloses the assumptions of the copier, who evidently did not deem it necessary to identify Geng Yan's full name because he assumed that the general's prowess as a healer was well-known to readers.

If indeed the official face of medicine was unmistakable to Sima Qian's audience and to ancient consumers of medical formulas, we must ask ourselves how the discrepancies between ancient and modern presentations of Chunyu Yi are to be explained. What accounts, in other words, for the modern propensity to see Chunyu Yi merely as a "doctor" and the Granary Master's records just as a medical text?

Certainly, it is tempting to chalk up the current view of Chunyu Yi to anachronism – the projection of modern categories back into the distant past. Yet anachronism does not tell us the whole story. The process by which the Granary Master was made into the physician Chunyu Yi began long before the twentieth century. By the Song dynasty, the bureaucratic resonances of the Granary Master's records of consultation were either lost or just overlooked. Instead, such records were largely read for clues about illness and therapy.[60] Take the case of Xu Shuwei 許叔微 (fl. AD 1132), the great medical authority and official.[61] In a chapter devoted to the subject of female ailments, Xu discussed illnesses stemming from celibacy in women, particularly Buddhist nuns and widows, who "suffer from desires that sprout but go unsatisfied." As Xu's remarks reveal, the existence of such ills was hotly debated in his time. In order to furnish proof of their existence, Xu cited one of the Granary Master's records of consultation, which, he reminded readers, contained the case of a female attendant who had fallen sick. As Xu further pointed out, the Granary Master had attributed the sickness to unfulfilled desires after examining her and noticing an irregular kidney pulse. By connecting the Granary Master's diagnosis to theories in Xu's time, this Song dynasty authority reasoned that the Granary Master had been aware of the adverse effects of celibacy.[62]

Xu's reading of the Granary Master's records is striking in its blatant disregard for the rhetorical and historical contexts that produced such records; it did not matter that Buddhist missionaries would not have arrived on the scene until centuries after Sima Qian's death, a fact Xu must have been aware of. In this regard, Xu's cavalier treatment of his sources stands in relief to those of his contemporaries, who were acutely aware that Sima Qian's retelling of the past had a purpose. Such contemporaries scrutinized the language and structure of the monumental history for clues as to the author's intent.[63] Xu, in contrast, seemed unconcerned with the larger political or moral resonances of the chapter. For him, the biography of the Granary Master was simply to be mined for "data." In this regard, Xu's interpretation of Sima Qian's biography of the Granary Master was hardly unique. By the Yuan 元 dynasty (1271–1368), the Granary Master's records circulated as an independent title,[64] suggesting that later medical authorities writing in the Yuan, Ming 明 (1368–1644), and Qing 清 (1644–1911) also emulated Xu's example in reading the records of consultation just as a guide for medical treatment. Like Xu, these later authors never breathed a word about the rhetorical function of Sima Qian's biography or the administrative practices that inspired the records. Instead, they took apart the contents of the biography in the *Records of the Grand Historian*, treating them as discrete parcels of information that could be rearranged around medical categories that would have been foreign to the original Han authors.[65]

None of this gets us any closer to learning *when* exactly the biography of the Granary Master and other early works were first read solely for their medical contents. In order to answer this question, we will have to know more about how early Chinese authors looked at the category of medicine. It will also be necessary to investigate when such authors began to lump the diverse arts of healing into a single category, a subject to which we turn in Chapter 4.

PART II

MEDICAL HISTORIES

4

LIU XIANG: THE IMPERIAL LIBRARY AND THE CREATION OF THE EXEMPLARY HEALER LIST

THUS FAR WE HAVE BEEN CONCERNED WITH THE personas of the medical fathers: the lore around them, the contexts in which such lore was created, and the processes by which it was converted into biographical information. What I have yet to show is who fused such lore into a single narrative about the genesis and history of the curative arts – in other words, who made the exemplary healer list? Toward this end, I investigate when historical narratives of medicine arose, which parties were responsible for writing such narratives, and what set of circumstances inspired these parties to take up the brush.

It would be worth saying something about the historical setting. The first three chapters of this book traced the making of exemplary medical personalities in the centuries leading up to and following the Han founding in 206 BC. This chapter will be different; the last years of the Former Han dynasty (206 BC–AD 9) in the late first century will serve as the backdrop. In the time of Chunyu Yi and Sima Qian, the Han house had vigorous rulers – rulers who pushed a powerful nomadic federation into the depths of Central Asia, seized lands from rebellious princes and greedy landlords, and castrated surly scribes (or so we are told). Yet by the end of the first century BC, the Liu house had lost much of its strength. According to traditional historians, a different constellation of colorful personalities dominated the court: sing-song girls who aspired to become consorts, child emperors, ambitious dowagers, and wicked uncles, to name a few. One wicked uncle, in particular, even managed to overthrow the Liu house and to establish the short-lived Xin 新 dynasty (AD 9–23) before a distant relative of the last Liu emperor founded his own dynasty known as the Later Han (AD 25–220). The precise reasons for the reversal of dynastic fortunes are disputed – though one would be well advised to steer clear of traditional explanations that chalk up the fall of the Han house to the sexual faults of rulers rather than to larger political or economic factors.

Although widely considered a period of political decline, the late first century BC was also an era of great intellectual ferment. Before an imperial relative usurped the Liu throne in AD 9, the reigns of the last Former Han emperors were marked by important achievements: the formation of a classical corpus, or the *Five Classics*; the emergence of scholastic lineages as a dominant force in the Chinese intellectual landscape; and new approaches to the interpretation of ancient texts. Last was the reorganization of the imperial collections, a massive undertaking not unlike the establishment of the library in Alexandria. Under the supervision of two imperial relatives, all manuscripts deemed to be of importance were collected, catalogued, and edited over two decades beginning in 26 BC. By the time the reorganization was completed, the imperial library collection of documents contained a subject catalogue for all texts.[1]

It was in this context of intellectual ferment that the exemplary healer list emerged, largely as a result of the initiative of Liu Xiang and his son Liu Xin 劉歆 (ca. 46 BC–AD 23), two major literati of the period. To show this, I ask when the authors of medical treatises and the practitioners of the curative arts began to look backward. I argue that a conception of medicine as an integrated art and subject of historical reflection emerged surprisingly late in early China. Early medical authors discussed specific techniques of healing and occasionally mentioned exemplary figures of the past. Yet it is no earlier than the third century AD – four hundred years *after* the earliest surviving medical manuscripts are dated – that the authors of medical treatises inserted exemplary healers into a narrative about the origins of medicine. Having traced the chronology of origins narratives, I then turn to the reasons why Huangfu Mi and other authors sought the roots of the curative arts. After considering different explanations, I demonstrate that the exemplary healer list was in fact Liu Xiang's creation. As the leader of the classicizing movement and the force behind the reorganization of the imperial collections, the imperial bibliographer was uniquely capable of bringing together miscellaneous strands of textual learning and lore about ancient healers. Although Liu Xiang was not a healer, the synthetic narrative that he composed supplied later authors of medical treatises with a template for writing about the history of the curative arts.

SETTING THE STAGE

As in previous chapters, the anonymously written manuscripts about healing will assume center stage in my story. At the same time, our discussion will also encompass works not concerned with healers or healing, including the ritual classics and etymological dictionaries of Han. Most important to our discussion, however, will be the subject catalogue that Liu Xiang produced during the reorganization of the imperial collections. Though no longer extant, scholars have reconstructed its contents from two later titles: the fragments of the *Seven Summaries* (*Qilüe* 七略) by Liu Xin, which was a revision of his father's preliminary catalogue, and the *Treatise on Arts and Literature* (*Yiwen zhi* 藝文志) by the Han chronicler Ban Gu 班固 (AD 32–92), which closely follows Liu Xin's *Seven Summaries*. The fact that the contents and wording of the two catalogues are virtually identical indicates that the younger Liu and Ban copied from Liu Xiang.

Our discussion will also bring attention to a new kind of medical work that emerged in the third century AD, compilations that bore the names of their authors. In contrast to earlier times, third-century readers associated works on the curative arts with historical authors named in prefaces. These include the *Treatise on Cold Damage Disorders and Various Illnesses* (*Shanghan zubing lun* 傷寒卒病論)[2] of Zhang Ji (AD 150–219); the *Classic of the Pulse* (*Maijing* 脈經) of the imperial medical attendant Wang Xi (third century AD), and the *AB Classic of the Yellow Emperor* (*Huangdi jiayi jing* 黃帝甲乙經; ca. AD 260) of Huangfu Mi.

One should *not* take the proliferation of manuscripts in early imperial China as a sign that readers acquired knowledge solely through reading. Up until the first centuries of Han, oral transmission represented a key facet of literate culture, a phenomenon explained by several different factors, including the physicality of the manuscripts. Writing had existed in China for more than a millennium before paper arrived on the scene. Invented in the first century AD by a court eunuch, paper technology was slow to be refined, and paper only became widely used in the post-Han period.[3] Prior to this time, copiers recorded manuscripts in heavier and more cumbersome mediums, like bamboo and wood, or silk, which, while neither heavy nor cumbersome, was rather expensive.[4] For these reasons, manuscripts tended to circulate within small, tight-knit communities of fathers and sons, or masters and disciples. The difficulty and expense of copying and memorizing texts furthermore discouraged prolific collecting and reading. "Given the slow pace of copying and memorizing in a manuscript culture largely dependent upon oral instruction," Michael Nylan writes, "the final authority of even the most renowned model and his writings could be trusted only insofar as circles of admirers committed themselves to preserving and transmitting their favorite texts."[5]

In addition, social practices of transmission also reinforced the primacy of orality, particularly before the time of Liu Xiang. In the early years of the empire, the transmission of texts generally occurred within the context of the relationship between a teacher and novice, or a father and son. The period of transmission was moreover an extended one. If one trusts the picture in the biography of the Granary Master, a teacher would first ascertain that the disciple was "the right person," meaning that the latter was of the requisite moral or personal qualities. Over the period of transmission, a teacher would not merely transfer the contents of a text but also initiate the novice into a way of understanding and using the text. In concrete terms, this meant that the novice would memorize the contents of the text and hear his teacher's explanations of it. Although novices also sometimes made written copies of the text, they assumed that the guidance of the teacher was essential for grasping the deeper meanings and application of the text, particularly ones attributed to ancient sages.[6] The dominance of textual initiation in early imperial China should be borne in mind, as it plays a central role in our story. As we shall see, Liu Xiang's challenge to this mode of textual transmission provided the catalyst for the writing of the first medical histories in China.

HISTORIES OF MEDICINE

To show Liu Xiang's hand in creating the earliest histories of medicine, we need to first demonstrate that such narratives were absent before his time. Toward this end, I return to the early corpus of medical manuscripts and treatises from the preimperial and early imperial periods. Through these methods, I reveal that authors only began to frame the various techniques of healing as a single art in the first century of our era. Only in the late second or third century AD do we begin to see these authors recounting the history of the healing arts through exemplary healers from antiquity.

The corpus of excavated documents from the late third and second centuries BC offers little evidence for origins narratives. Take the manuals recovered from two tombs, Zhangjiashan (ca. 186 BC) and Mawangdui (ca. 168 BC). Unlike the earlier Guanju manuscript, the authors of these works actually referred to exemplary figures by name (see Chapter 2). The author of the *Pulling Book* (see Chapter 2), which set forth directions for therapeutic stretches and breathing exercises, mentioned in passing one Ancestor Peng (Pengzu 彭祖), a figure renowned for his longevity;[7] the author of the famous sexual cultivation text from Mawangdui also opened with comments from the Yellow Emperor and other mythical figures of high antiquity.[8] These brief glimpses provided *no* explanation as to how such figures were connected to contemporary healers – or, for that matter – any other exemplary healers. Further, the authors revealed nothing about the genesis of medicine or the contributions of such figures to medical knowledge. As a result, one might say that the early manuscripts merely supplied the material for histories of medicine but not actual histories.

A historical recollection of medicine is absent even from the "Biographies of Bian Que and the Granary Master" (see Chapters 2 and 3). This chapter in the *Records of the Grand Historian* contains information that scholars would later use to construct medical histories, for it mentions masters and ancient exemplary healers. Sima Qian, for example, revealed the name of Bian Que's master, a divine being who bestowed upon him a magical potion to see through solid objects.[9] In his description of Bian Que's encounter with a patient, Sima Qian referred to another ancient figure, Yufu 俞跗, "who was able to treat illnesses without the use of medicinal decoctions, sweet and warm wines, stone needles, raising and pulling exercises, massage therapy for calibrating the blood and vessels, or application of heat and drugs."[10] Similarly, Sima Qian explained the Granary Master's association with two contemporaries who instructed him in the curative arts, Gongsun Guang 公孫光 and Yang Qing. At one point during the biography, Yang Qing presented the Granary Master with his secret formulas and works of supposedly ancient provenance after verifying that the latter was in fact the "right person."[11]

Despite its resemblance to later histories and origins narratives, Sima Qian's chapter about the pair did not represent a history of medicine so much as a biography of two men who practiced healing. As Jin Shiqi points out, the very title of the chapter ("The Biographies of Bian Que and the Granary Master") alerts us to the fact that medicine was not Sima Qian's main subject. Crucially, Sima Qian chose to entitle the chapter something other than the "Biography of Healers" even though both Bian Que and the Granary Master were famous for their curative prowess. Titling a chapter "The Biography of Healers" would *not* have been out of the question, because the *Records of the Grand Historian* has chapters with analogous titles: "The Biographies of the Hemerologists" (*Rizhe liezhuan* 日者列傳), the "Biographies of the Diviners" (*Guice liezhuan* 龜策列傳), or the "Biographies of the Classicists" (*Rulin liezhuan* 儒林列傳).[12]

What is more, Jin Shiqi's observations highlight how inappropriate it would be to read the chapter about Bian Que and the Granary Master as an early history of medicine. For example, Sima Qian did not offer anything in the vein of general reflections on medicine, aside from a passing comment that Bian Que was associated with the art of taking the pulse.[13] In other words, Sima did not insert Bian Que and the Granary Master into a general narrative regarding the origins and history of the medical arts. For example, the historian brought up Yufu in the biography of Bian Que, but Bian Que in this instance specifically denied any connection to Yufu. Similarly, the Granary Master mentioned works attributed to Bian Que and the Yellow Emperor. Yet, as Donald Harper points out, the Granary Master professed to know nothing about the teachers of his own masters. Consequently, it is impossible to trace several generations of continuous transmission, let alone reconstruct any relationship between Bian Que and the Granary Master.[14]

Sima Qian's omission of any story about the genesis and history of medicine in the "Biographies of Bian Que and the Granary Master" is all the more striking, when one compares it to another chapter of the *Records of the Grand Historian*, the "Biography of the Classicists." In the latter, Sima Qian provided an origins story for classics and other important forms of ancient wisdom in the decline of the Zhou 周 royal house (ca. eleventh century – 221 BC) and Confucius's dissatisfaction with his age. Although Sima Qian stopped short of tracing continuous lines of textual filiation from Confucius to Sima Qian's time, his account nevertheless described the key figures among the seventy disciples of Confucius. It briefly related the careers of the leading exemplars of ancient learning in the centuries leading up to unification and then named the chief custodians of ancient learning in the Han.[15] Nothing of this sort can be found in the "Biographies of Bian Que and the Granary Master." In the latter, Sima Qian entirely refrained from recounting how medicine came into being or even putting into a single category the teachers of Bian Que and the Granary Master, on the one hand, and the ancient sages, on the other.

The *Inner Classic* (see Chapter 2) also provides little evidence that the authors imagined the curative arts in historical terms. To be sure, figures of purported antiquity appeared throughout this text – for example, the author showed the Yellow Emperor conversing with his teacher about therapeutic principles.[16] There are, moreover, references to nameless ancient figures: to the sages of old or the perfected men of the highest antiquity.[17] In one passage, the author even credited unnamed sages with discovering the key features of the body.[18] Yet none of this added up to an origins narrative. Though the *Inner Classic* treated the various techniques of healing as transmitted knowledge and stressed the importance of initiation by a master, the authors made no effort to supply names of great healers or medical progenitors.[19] The reader, for example, is never afforded a glimpse of textual transmission beyond a single generation. In addition, the discussions of antiquity did little to give the impression of the curative arts in time. In many cases the authors entirely omitted the names of exemplars, ancient or recent. What is more, such authors used descriptions of the past to emphasize the gulf between the practices of the past and those of the present.[20]

The relative inattention to the history of the curative arts makes sense; medical authors of the second and third centuries BC did not lump the various techniques of diagnosis or healing into a single, catchall category.[21] Instead, authors in that era referred to healing in terms of specific techniques and most often separately: the way of pulse diagnosis (*xiangmai zhi dao* 相脈之道),[22] the medicaments (*duyao* 毒藥), moxa (*jiubing* 灸炳), stone needles (*bianshi* 砭石), the way or method of needling (*zhendao* 針道 or *zhenfa* 針法), and pulling and massage exercises (*daoyin anqiao* 導引按蹻).[23]

In addition, preimperial authors used the term *yi* to refer to *attendants* charged with looking after the various physical needs of others. This sense of the term was broader than its later usages: after the second century AD, the authors of etymological dictionaries treated *yi* as synonymous with *healers* as "*yi* were craftsmen who controlled ailments" (*zhibing gong* 治病工).[24] In contrast, preimperial authors sometimes used *yi* in the more general sense of someone who attended to the diverse facets of the body's upkeep. When discussing the organizing of the palace bureaus, the author of the utopian *Rites of Zhou* (*Zhouli* 周禮), which may date to the late Warring States, alluded to the various *yi*: the "*yi* of beasts" (*shouyi* 獸醫), the "*yi* of illnesses" (*jiyi* 疾醫), the "*yi* of sores" (*yangyi* 瘍醫), and the "*yi* of foodstuff" (*shiyi* 食醫), all of whom were under the direction of the "master *yi*" (*yishi* 醫師). What catches the eye here is the reference to the "*yi* of foodstuff," which the author explained as the attendants charged with selecting and preparing the ruler's meals and drinks.[25] Authors of Qin and early Former Han texts moreover kept with this habit of using *yi* to describe attendants of various kinds, like the woman who attended the nurses of imperial children (*ruyi* 乳醫).[26] Echoes of the early practice of differentiating between various attendants can be found in the biography of Bian Que. There, Sima Qian mentioned that the legendary healer was referred to by different names: as the "*yi* for ailments below the belt" (*daixia yi* 帶下醫) (i.e., for women), the "*yi* for the eyes and ears, and for paralysis" (*ermu bi yi* 耳目痹醫), and the "*yi* for children" (*xiao er yi* 小兒醫).[27]

It is not until the *Inner Classic*, compiled in the first century BC or AD, that we catch the glint of a notion of medicine as a singular art. Chapter 75 of this text mentioned the "way of the *yi*" (*yidao* 醫道; *yi zhi dao* 醫之道) twice in passing.[28] However suggestive, such phrases rarely appeared in the *Inner Classic* – a dearth also present in texts such as the *Divine Husbandman's Classic of Pharmacopeia* (*Shennong bencao jing* 神農本草經) and the *Classic of Problems* (*Nanjing* 難經), all typically dated to the first century AD. Most often, the *Inner Classic* conformed to the earlier practice of discussing specific techniques. Chapter 12 presents one such example, as it is devoted entirely to describing the various forms of therapy: the administration of medicaments, application of heat and fire, needling, pulling, and massage. Though collected together in one chapter, the different techniques of healing, the author emphasized, had diverse origins. The practice of using fine needles, for example, originated in the south, whereas the medicaments (*duyao*) were inventions of the West, and so forth.[29] Most tellingly, the author never used the word *yi* once in Chapter 12, which suggests that he had yet to take the final step to lump all of the therapeutic methods under a single category. Indeed, in his final comment, he highlighted the diversity of such methods: "The sage combines the *sundry* (*za* 雜) in treating, obtaining what is fitting for each case, and in using different methods, the ills are all cured."[30]

Early medical authors only began to consistently put the various curative techniques into the same category after the late second or early third century AD. The preface to the *Cold Damage Disorders* is one of the earliest potential texts to treat medicine in such terms. I say *potential* because the provenance of the preface, traditionally attributed to Zhang Ji, is uncertain (on this point, see Chapter 6). If we momentarily bracket the matter of its provenance, the preface suggests several things about how authors conceived of the curative arts in the last years of Han. To begin with, the author used a two-character combination, *yiyao* 醫藥, to speak of the curative arts. In doing so, he broke with the earlier practice of classifying the various curative arts according to specific techniques. Instead, this author acknowledged that all of the different techniques constituted healing, and he conflated healing with diagnosis.[31]

The new way of thinking about the various techniques of therapy and healing as an integrated art is evident from two works dating to the third century: the *Classic of the Pulse* by the imperial medical attendant Wang Xi and the *AB Classic* by Huangfu Mi. While reflecting upon the risks of therapies, Wang Xi wrote in his preface, "The deployment of the arts of healing and medicaments (*yiyao*) is linked with matters of life and death."[32] As Wang Xi was concerned here with the difficulties of pulse diagnosis, his term *yiyao* encompassed diagnostic practices as well as therapy. Similarly, in the opening sentence to the *AB Classic*, Huangfu Mi spoke of the ancient roots of the "Way of Medicine," and in the next breath explained the origins of medicaments and decoctions, pulse diagnosis, techniques for observing the appearance, and acupuncture needles.[33] Taken together, the remarks by Wang Xi and Huangfu Mi indicate that by the third century, authors commonly subsumed the diverse techniques of prognosis and healing under a single rubric.

Besides framing diagnosis and therapy as a unified art, the authors of medical treatises from the third century also began to look back at the history of curative arts. The author to the preface to the *Cold Damage Disorders* – which scholars often treat as a work of the third century – traced the history of the arts by reciting a list of exemplary figures: "In high antiquity there were the Divine Husbandman and the Yellow Emperor, Qibo 岐伯, Bogao 伯高, Lord Thunder, Shaoyu 少俞, Shaoshi 少師, and Zhongwen 仲文." Many of these legendary culture heroes appeared in earlier texts, the manuscripts recovered from the Mawangdui site and the *Inner Classic*, for example. Yet unlike earlier works, this author traced the history of the curative arts through successive periods: "In middle antiquity there was Lord Changsang 長桑 (i.e., the teacher of Bian Que) and Bian Que, and in the Han there was Yang Qing, (i.e., the teacher of the Granary Master) of the eighth order of honor, and the Granary Master."[34]

This impulse to think of the curative arts in historical terms was broadly shared among medical authors of the third century. The author of the *Classic of the Pulse*, Wang Xi looked back upon his predecessors with an esteem that verged on veneration. He praised Bian Que and Attendant He for their prowess as healers. He also singled out Zhang Ji for his "clear-sighted" investigations of illness and thorough prognoses: "If there was the slightest doubt, Zhang Ji would investigate matters in search of verification." Other comments by Wang Xi reveal that he saw the curative arts in terms of a long history, as when he declared, "At this time I have selected and collected the works of authors from Qibo to Hua Tuo, their classics, discourses, essentials, and judgments, and combined them into a work of ten rolls." As some of the figures mentioned by Wang Xi may be unfamiliar, it is worth highlighting the span of time that separated Qibo from Hua Tuo (d. ca. AD 208). Presumably a contemporary of the legendary Yellow Emperor, Qibo was a figure of high antiquity, whereas Hua Tuo had died only decades before Wang composed the *Classic of the Pulse*.[35]

It is Huangfu Mi who wrote the fullest account of medical history. Given its central importance to our story, it is worth looking at an extended excerpt:

> 夫醫道 所興, 其來久矣。上古神農始嘗草木而知百藥。黃帝咨訪岐伯、伯高、少俞之徒, 內考五藏(臟)六腑, 外綜經絡血氣色候, 參之天地, 驗之人物, 本性命, 窮神極變, 而鍼道生焉。其論至妙, 雷公受業傳之於後, 伊尹以亞聖之才, 撰用《神農本草》, 以為《湯液》。中古名醫,有俞跗、醫緩、扁鵲,秦有醫和,漢有倉公,其論皆經理識本, 非徒胗 (診)病而已。漢有張仲景, 華佗[36]奇方異治, 施 世者多,亦不能盡記其本末。
>
> It has been a long time since the Way of Medicine arose. In high antiquity, the Divine Husbandman first tasted the plants and thereby learned of the properties of the myriad medicines. Consulting with the likes of Qibo, Bogao, and Shaoyu, the Yellow Emperor inspected the five *yin* and six *yang* visceral systems within the body and synthesized the vessels and collateral vessels, blood, *qi*, appearance, and indicators without. All these were examined in light of the conditions of Heaven and Earth, verified with respect to humans and beasts, and rooted in the different natures; once the mysteries and transformations had been exhaustively interrogated, the way of needling came into being. The analyses were of the utmost subtlety. Lord Thunder inherited this enterprise and transmitted it to later men. Possessing the abilities of a secondary sage, Yi Yin [i.e., the minister to the Shang dynasty founders] (trad. 17th c. BC) edited the *Divine Husbandman's Classic of Pharmacopeia* to create the text called the *Decoctions* (*Tangye* 湯液).
>
> Among the famed healers of middle antiquity were Yufu, Attendant Huan, and Bian Que. The Qin had Attendant He, and the Han the Granary Master. Their analyses captured root principles and thus they did far more than just examine the ill. During the Han, there was also Zhang Zhongjing [i.e., Zhang Ji] and Hua Tuo, who used extraordinary formulas and unusual treatments. Although there were many who

disseminated their teachings to the world, the works of these figures have not been recorded completely.[37]

Several points are worth drawing out from this account. To begin with, its derivative quality deserves mention. Most of the figures mentioned by Huangfu Mi appeared in earlier sources that survive to this day. The episode about Attendant He surfaced in sources of the Warring States, and tales about Bian Que and the Granary Master were collected in the *Records of the Grand Historian* (see Chapters 2 and 3). Even the claim advanced by Huangfu Mi regarding the Divine Husbandman's hand in the creation of medicine was less original than it would initially seem. A similar description showed up in the *Master Huainan* (*Huainanzi* 淮南子), a classic of persuasion compiled around 139 BC.[38] What *was* novel about Huangfu Mi's account was the way that he brought together representations of healers and innovators spread out between a variety of texts and genres.

Its derivative nature aside, Huangfu Mi's account is especially noteworthy on a second count, in that it may be thought of as an origins narrative.[39] Here, Huangfu Mi attempted to explain the genesis of medical knowledge, which he thought did not develop overnight but over innumerable generations. The Divine Husbandman had illuminated the power of medicinal herbs; the Yellow Emperor and his interlocutors had discovered the key features of the human body, knowledge necessary for the practice of acupuncture; and the sagely minister Yi Yin had edited the *Divine Husbandman's Classic of Pharmacopeia*. The creation of medical knowledge did not end in high antiquity, however. According to Huangfu Mi, subsequent figures elaborated upon the insights of earlier healers and progenitors. The Granary Master's conceptions of the body, he wrote, were rooted in the learning of the *Basic Questions* (*Suwen* 素問), a work of presumably high antiquity. In the third century AD, Zhang Ji "expanded upon the decoctions of Yi Yin" to compose a treatise on medicaments, and Wang Xi subsequently rearranged the treatise by Zhang Ji to make it more accessible.[40]

MATTERS OF TIMING

The foregoing discussion leaves us wondering why authors of the third century AD, unlike their predecessors, conceived of healing as an integrated art and outfitted it with an origins narrative. To this end, a review of competing hypotheses shall help us determine the most plausible scenario: that the creation of an exemplary healer list owed much to the activities of Liu Xiang. Although Liu Xiang worked with the imperial medical attendant Li Zhuguo 李柱國 (fl. ca. 26 BC), it was Liu Xiang and not the medical attendant who was in a unique position to pull together the specific list of exemplary healers. This is because Liu Xiang's position as the imperial bibliographer afforded him access to obscure texts that would otherwise have been inaccessible. Additionally, Liu Xiang's leadership in the classicizing movement, explained below, gave him both the wherewithal and the confidence to interpret and reconstruct a wide variety of ancient works that most of his contemporaries would have shied away from.

Although many of the elements in origins narratives existed long before Huangfu Mi, there is reason to believe that earlier authors living in the second century BC could not have invented the present list of exemplary healers. For a start, most of the reflections on the origins and evolution of medicine surface in prefaces that appeared after the second century AD. Yet prefaces – reflecting complex notions of authorship – were not at all common before the end of the first century BC; only after the late Former Han did writers make a habit of identifying their authorship in prefaces, expressing their hopes for a good reputation among posterity.[41]

In addition, early medical authors would have had difficulty laying their hands on texts that supplied much information about figures from the preimperial period. For example, the *Tradition of Zuo*, which preserved the fullest and earliest surviving account of Attendant He, did not circulate widely until the late first century BC. It was already late in the Former Han dynasty by the time the son of the imperial bibliographer promoted the text in the capital.[42] Nor did the *Records of the Grand Historian*, an important source of information for authors of the third century AD, circulate widely before late Former Han. Deposited in imperial archives for the perusal of rulers and their trusted advisors, the *Records of the Grand Historian* languished away, largely unknown to the literate elite.[43] The fate of the *Records of the Grand Historian* was far from an isolated occurrence. As Michael Nylan explains, many of the texts that contain information about earlier figures like Bian Que and Attendant He had limited circulation. Before the late first century BC, many preimperial manuscripts were kept in the personal libraries of Han princes and rulers. The uncle of an emperor of the second century BC held a library that boasted of the best editions of older texts, an example that spurred his nephew to follow in his footsteps. Yet the existence of such libraries did little to broaden the horizons of even elite readers. The emperor was known to guard access to his collection jealously, even going so far as to deny entry to an imperial prince.[44]

In the unlikely event that the men of the second century BC had access to many old manuscripts, it was far from a foregone conclusion that they would have culled such works for clues about the origins of medicine. As Nylan shows, at the end of the first century BC even the most educated men in the realm found it difficult to decode old texts written in the archaic scripts of the preimperial period.[45] Moreover, many educated members of the Former Han elite still believed that understanding old texts required the guidance of a master,[46] and healers were no exception. In his response to court queries, the Granary Master emphasized the importance of being initiated by a teacher into the arts: he only became a successful healer once he found a teacher who could explain the larger import of medical texts, and his biography revealed how crucial his teacher's explanations were to grasping the proper applications of drug formulas and other forms of therapy.[47] As Nathan Sivin writes, the biography of the Granary Master betrays the belief that "the truths were too deeply embedded in these texts" and that "in the degenerate present only those initiated by a master could hope to comprehend them."[48]

All this raises the question of what drove the later transformations in conceptions of healing. What specifically had changed in the centuries between Chunyu Yi and Huangfu Mi? One possibility is that the origins narratives in Huangfu Mi's day reflected the emergence of medical lineages. By lineages, I mean the exclusive multigenerational networks of masters and disciples that traced continuous lines of textual filiation from an apical figure.

The aforementioned possibility is worth taking seriously. At the very least, it is consistent with recent scholarship on early China. In contrast to older work,[49] such scholarship emphasizes the ways in which the social practice of transmission changed over the course of the Han period.[50] In the early Han, the relationship between master and student, though highly ritualized, was fluid, nonexclusive, and open ended. Like the Granary Master, a man could study with more than one teacher over his lifetime. Similarly, a teacher would initiate his disciples into a wide variety of texts associated with disparate figures. This much is suggested by the biography of the Granary Master, where Sima Qian wrote that the early Han figure had received a number of texts from his master, including those attributed to Bian Que and the Yellow Emperor.[51] Or, as

Michael Nylan points out, the process of initiation was not necessarily focused on textual transmission. A master might teach his disciples a set of technical skills, or even a "powerful way of interacting with the world" encapsulated in a text.[52]

By the end of the first century AD, however, the practice of initiation changed significantly. To begin with, the relationship between master and disciple acquired a new permanence, as such a relationship was now embedded in a broader network of men, or a scholastic lineage. Modeled directly after the patrilineal family, the scholastic lineage spanned many generations and purported to transmit particular interpretations of classics originating from a founding patriarch. Over the first century AD, membership in an established lineage became essential for acquiring a foothold into the bureaucracy as it represented an important determinant of scholastic authority. Given the stakes, it is unsurprising that the imperial state regulated the relationship between members of lineages. The state required that pupils register under their teachers and made them liable to punishment under statutes mandating collective responsibility.[53]

There are reasons not to chalk up the emergence of origins narratives to the rise of medical lineages. Huangfu's origins narrative contained few indications that the third-century literatus saw himself on a direct line of transmission from antiquity. Huangfu Mi *did* state that Lord Thunder inherited the "enterprise" from the Yellow Emperor and transmitted it to later people. But any talk of transmission ended there. More seriously, Huangfu Mi said nothing about his personal connection to any of these figures or the circumstances in which he came to possess such revelations. Did a master initiate him into the mysteries of the medical classics? Or did he perhaps discover the revelations in one of the bookshops in the capital, which, in the first century AD, were just starting to crop up. Huangfu Mi's silence about his relationship to antiquity is suggestive.[54] Had he told the history of medicine to prove his membership in a scholastic lineage, one would expect him to have said something about how he was related to a founding patriarch.

There is another reason why the rise of scholastic lineages does not explain the emergence of medical histories in early China. A comparison of sources in the centuries before and after the first century AD – the moment at which scholastic lineages emerged suddenly as a force to be reckoned with – reveals no obvious differences in the transmission of medical knowledge from the Former Han dynasty (see Table 5). In fact, the relationships between masters and disciples who lived after the first

Table 5 *Representations of Master-Disciple Clusters*

	Master	Dates	Disciple	Source	Notes
1	Gongsun Guang	Ca. 180 BC	Chunyu Yi	*Shiji*, 105.2815	
2	Yang Qing	Ca. 180 BC	Chunyu Yi	*Shiji*, 105.2815; 2796	
3	Chunyu Yi	Fl. Ca. 180 BC	Du Xin 杜信, Gao Qi 高期, Feng Xin 馮信, Song Yi 宋邑, Tang An 唐安, Wang Yu 王禹	*Shiji*, 105.2816–17	
4	Fu Weng 涪翁 or the Old Man of the Fu River		Cheng Gao 程高	*Hou Hanshu*, 82/72B.2735	Hagiographical account (the Old Man resembles an adept)
5	Li Shaojun 李少君		Ji Liao 薊遼 (fl. Later Han) or Ji Zixun 薊子訓	*Shenxian zhuan jiaoshi*, 264	Li Shaojun lived centuries before Ji Liao
6	Zhang Bozu 張伯祖	Late second century	Zhang Ji	*Yi shuo*, 1/14a	References to Zhang Bozu emerge very late
7	Zhang Ji	Late second century and early third century	Du Du 杜度 and Wei Fan 衛汎	*Yi shuo*, 1/14a *Taiping yulan*, 722/3329a	References to Zhang Ji's disciples are very late
8	Hua Tuo	D. ca. AD 208	Li Dangzhi 李當之, Wu Pu 吳普, and Fan A 樊阿	*Hou Hanshu*, 82/72B.2739–40; *Sanguo zhi*, 29.804, *Yi shuo*, 1/14b	Hagiographical account; Hua Tuo and his disciples were purportedly adepts who lived into their hundreds
9	Wang Heping 王和平	Fl. ca. AD 180	Sun Yong 孫邕 and Xia Rong 夏榮	*Hou Hanshu*, 82/72B.2751, *Sanguo zhi*, 29.805	Wang Heping was purportedly an immortal
10	Cheng Gao 程高	First century AD	Guo Yu 郭玉	*Hou Hanshu*, 82/72B.2735	Hagiographical elements; see the entry for Fu Weng

century AD are indistinguishable from the ones described by Sima Qian. As before, such relationships were confined to two generations.

To explain the rise of origins narratives, we are better served by shifting our attention away from scholastic lineages to the classicizing movement. Before going too much further, it is necessary to say something more about the latter's major players and motivations. At the center of this movement were two blood relatives of the emperor, Liu Xiang and his son Liu Xin. Besides leading the reorganization of the imperial collections, Liu Xiang and his son wrote about an array of subjects, including the classics, the education of women, the lives of immortals, history, alchemy, and astrology. They also left their mark when they began to promote their vision of the classical past. In the late first century the Lius embraced the idea that it was possible to bypass long-standing oral traditions in order to understand the contents of ancient classics, believed to contain the revelations of sages.[55] This was a radical idea, one that represented nothing less than an attack on the court-appointed Academicians, a group that enshrined the practice of textual initiation by a master. Ostensibly, the Lius justified such an attack on the grounds that the Academicians and the practice of initiation not only failed to produce men of insight into the Way, but also obscured the true meaning of classical authors. In the process of transmitting texts from one generation to the next, Liu and his group charged, the Academicians had introduced errors into the classics. To them, it was better for someone to interpret directly the relics or textual remnants of the sages. Moreover, this coterie developed word lists and lexicons, which facilitated the deciphering of unfamiliar texts written in regional dialects or archaic scripts.[56]

With this idea, Liu Xiang and the members of his circle devoted their energies to creating critical editions from pre- and early imperial materials and bringing attention to long-neglected texts. One such text, the *Stratagems of the Warring States* (see Chapter 2), offered surviving accounts of Bian Que that probably predated those found in the *Records of the Grand Historian*. Another, the *Tradition of Zuo*, which contained the fullest description of Attendant He, was rescued from virtual obscurity and popularized by Liu Xin. The same group of bibliophiles was instrumental in bringing attention to important recent works with medical content. For example, Liu Xiang and his protégé's admiration for the *Records of the Grand Historian* led them to portray it as a model of historical writing, which increased its prominence.[57] All this opened the thinking of later medical authors to more sophisticated concepts of a medical narrative than had been apparent to the authors of the second or third centuries BC.

The medical prefaces of the second and third centuries AD bear testimony to the influence of the classicizing movement, as they reveal that the authors saw old medical works as the relics of sagely revelation. Like Liu Xiang, they not only believed that they could reconstruct old texts but also felt it incumbent on them to do so. The author of the *Classic of the Pulse*, Wang Xi, saw his contribution in terms of a larger project of textual restoration: "The texts transmitted from the sages are mysterious, and so over the ages few practitioners have been able to employ them." Wang Xi's complaints about the incoherence of transmitted texts should be taken with a grain of salt. Evidently, he believed that by collating different editions of texts, he would secure for himself a place in "the lineup of ancient worthies."[58]

The influence of the classicizing movement is most marked in the works of Huangfu Mi, whose career as an esteemed scholar and healer is discussed in the final chapter. Like Wang Xi, Huangfu Mi underscored the corrupt and fragmentary state of purportedly old medical works: "At present," he wrote, "there are the *Classic of the Needle* (*Zhenjing* 鍼道) in nine rolls, the *Basic Questions* in nine rolls, and the 298 rolls that make up the *Inner Classic*." Yet such works, he further noted, were hardly usable: "Parts have also been lost, and so even where the analyses are far-reaching, relating a great many things, they are of little practical use; and much of the text is jumbled." Such problems notwithstanding, Huangfu Mi asserted that by sifting through the textual remnants of the sages, the original sequence and wording of the classics could be restored by discerning readers such as he. Because the format as well as the content of such texts embodied the sage's understanding of the body, Huangfu Mi believed that his exegetical efforts would clarify the underlying principles of medicine.[59]

The Lius' reorganization of the imperial library, closely related to the classicizing movement, also proved instrumental to the development of medical histories in China. Not only did Liu Xiang and his circle create definitive editions of the technical literature, including the medical arts (not to mention the *Five Classics* and other important works of the preimperial period), they also made a subject catalogue for all items in the imperial library, including one for the medical corpus (*yijing* 醫經).[60] With the assistance of the imperial medical attendant, Liu Xiang collected and catalogued works broadly concerned with diagnosis and therapy.

The influence of the Lius on later authors is evident from the way that the authors subsumed the curative arts under the rubric of *yi*. Based on the *Seven Summaries* and the *Treatise on Arts and Literature*, it seems that the Lius may have been some of the very first authors to use *yi* to mean "diagnosis and therapy" in general. In this respect, the Lius anticipated Huangfu Mi's broad usage of the term. They did, however, place drug formulas in a related but separate category.[61] Neither the Lius nor Ban Gu provided a rationale for listing the cardinal formulas separately from the classics of *yi*. Judging from surviving manuscripts dating from the Former Han dynasty, the separate designation probably reflected the tendency for works on formulas to circulate as independent texts. Still, the fact that the Lius associated the categories of formulas with the classics of *yi* is evident from several features: in both catalogues, they put the cardinal formulas immediately after the classics of *yi*, and their complaints about "middling healers" indicate that the cardinal formulas were one of the resources to heal the body.

Regardless of how the Lius categorized the formulas, the *Seven Summaries* and the *Treatise on Arts and Literature* bore witness to the expanding scope of *yi*, a development that anticipated Huangfu Mi's usage of the term. In both of these catalogues, the Lius described *yi* as a range of diagnostic and curative techniques, as in the following excerpt:

> 醫經者, 原人血脈經 (絡) 〔落〕骨髓陰陽表裏, 以起百病之本, 死生之分, 而用度箴石湯火所施, 調百藥齊和之所宜。 至齊之得, 猶慈石取鐵, 以物相使。拙者失理, 以瘉爲劇, 以生爲死。

> The various classics of medicine investigate the blood and vessels, bones and marrow, *yin* and *yang*, and the outer and inner regions of man; they illuminate the roots of the myriad illnesses and the boundaries between life and death, so as to list the proper applications of the needles, decoctions, and heat, and to calibrate the proper mixtures of the myriad medicaments and dosages. All these cause the body to reach its equilibrium, much like magnets attracting iron; this is to use substances to activate one another. But the unskillful healer (*yi*) will lose sight of the larger pattern of the illness, mistaking the sick who can be healed with those suffering from irremediable illnesses, and those that will live with those who will die.[62]

Note that in this passage the Lius brought all of the disparate therapies together under the single rubric *yi*. The Lius and Ban had concluded that the *yi* corpus, in spite of its diversity, was integrated in contents and aims.

The Lius anticipated Huangfu Mi's conception of medicine in another way: in the process of reorganizing the imperial collection, they included the earliest surviving list of exemplary healers. In this connection, consider the following excerpt from the *Seven Summaries* and the *Treatise on Arts and Literature*:

> 太古有岐伯、俞拊 (跗), 中世有扁鵲、秦和, 蓋論病以及國, 原診以知政。漢興有倉公。今其技術晻昧, 故論其書, 以序方技為四種。
>
> In high antiquity, there were Qibo and Yufu; in middle antiquity, there were Bian Que and He of Qin, whose analyses of illnesses had implications for the state and who examined the ill to learn the circumstances of governance. Since the founding of Han, there has been the Granary Master. At present the arts have fallen into obscurity, and for this reason we have analyzed the documents, ordering the arts into four kinds.[63]

In the preceding text we see that the Lius and Ban charted the progress of medicine from high antiquity to their own times, through the middle of the Spring and Autumn (771–453 BC) to the recent past. Naturally, they were not the first to mention very early healers. As previously discussed, earlier works, such as the Mawangdui manuscripts from the early Han or the *Records of the Grand Historian*, contained isolated references to mythical healers such as Yufu or Bian Que. In contrast to earlier works, however, which made only passing reference to exemplary healers, Liu Xiang wove various strands of legends and persons (real or mythical) together in a single coherent narrative history of medicine.

The fact that the Lius' origins narrative drew from such a wide range of sources, including historical chronicles, deserves attention. Take Liu's invocation of Attendant He, who was unlikely to have been a household name; Attendant He's name appeared only in two historical chronicles of the preimperial period, and these, as we saw previously, did not circulate widely. It is thus unlikely that many people before the late first century BC connected this figure to a larger history of medicine. The decision on the part of the Lius and Ban to separate time into the three discrete stages of high antiquity, middle antiquity, and the recent past furnished the prototype for Huangfu Mi's list of exemplary healers. Moreover, Huangfu's preface closely followed Liu Xin's account. What is more, Huangfu Mi acknowledged his debt to Liu Xin in an explicit fashion: "I have followed the text of the *Seven Summaries*, the *Treatise on Arts and Literature,* and the eighteen-roll version of the *Inner Classic*."[64]

CONCLUSION AND DISCUSSION

The practice of composing lists of exemplary healers and tracing the history of medicine originated with Liu Xiang. In many regards, Liu Xiang's list of exemplary healers represented a major change in the way that the literati approached the curative arts. While previous authors had written about therapy and diagnosis for centuries before Liu Xiang, they did not commonly articulate how such techniques originated in antiquity, nor did they possess the kind of origins narrative that Huangfu Mi wrote in the third century AD. In contrast, Liu Xiang was in a unique position to bring together disparate legends and textual fragments into a historical sequence. Unlike earlier healers and medical authors, Liu Xiang had access to obscure manuscripts that contained the pieces of legends that would later become standard fare in historical narratives about medicine. And unlike the imperial medical attendant who assisted him in reorganizing the medical corpus, Liu Xiang was both inclined to and capable of scouring such ancient works for clues about the genesis of the curative arts. As the leaders of the classicizing movement, Liu Xiang and his son created the tools to bypass long-standing modes of oral transmission to interpret the sage's relics directly.

It remains to say a word about where the arguments of this chapter sit within the larger book. The first three chapters showed the arbitrariness of classifying stories about Attendant He and other ancient exemplars as medical history. Such stories, I argued, originally bore only a tangential relationship to the concerns of healers, as they were made by unrelated parties and for a variety of ends. In this chapter, I demonstrate that the act of placing such materials in the category of medical history was not the work of twentieth-century scholars like Needham. On the contrary, the process of extracting such stories from their original contexts and converting them into sources of medical history began in the Han. This process was sparked by the efforts of the imperial bibliographer, who systematized and overhauled the knowledge of his day.

Huangfu Mi was hardly the last author before Needham to recite the names and deeds of exemplary healers. Such a practice was in fact ubiquitous in Chinese medical culture before the twentieth century. Found in medieval manuscripts containing drug formulas, printed prefaces explaining the rationales of treatises in the eleventh and twelfth centuries, and the biographies of medical personalities of late imperial China, the list of ancient exemplars was invoked by later healers and medical authors, who sang the praises and recited the accomplishments of bygone men in order to illuminate the Way of Medicine. Indeed, the importance of the past to medicine's identity was signaled by the placement of Huangfu Mi's list of ancient figures on the entrance to the sixteenth-century College of Imperial Healers, where it was emblazoned. By the sixteenth century, however, the list of exemplars was longer and the lore about predecessors richer than in Huangfu Mi's day.[65] Huangfu Mi was now even included among their ranks.

How did the list of exemplary healers endure over the centuries? Needless to say, much had happened between Huangfu Mi's time and the sixteenth century. The intervening centuries witnessed important developments, such as the advent of official medicine in Tang; the influx of foreign medicine, including varieties brought in from India; and the changes in medical organization, the emergence of scholastic lineages modeled after a Neo-Confucian counterpart, in particular.[66] Given all this, the burden lies with the historian to explain how Huangfu Mi's list persisted over so many centuries. So we turn next to the subsequent incarnations of the list during China's long medieval period.

5

ZHANG JI: THE KALEIDOSCOPIC FATHER

AT THE CLOSE OF CHAPTER 4, WE ESTABLISHED THAT Huangfu Mi's list of exemplary healers endured for centuries. How do we come to understand that, despite disparate outward manifestations in varying time periods, we always return to the same list of ancient fathers? Is it safe to assume that the portraits of the medical fathers remained static through the centuries after Huangfu Mi? Or did the archive evolve over China's medieval period, and if so, by what means?

For answers to these questions, I examine the shifting representations of Zhang Ji (ca. AD 150–219),[1] a figure found among the ranks of Huangfu Mi's exemplary healers and Needham's medical fathers. By all accounts, Zhang Ji was a figure of unrivaled importance to the classical medical tradition. Regarded by later healers as the ancestor of all drug formulary, Zhang Ji invites comparisons to the Roman physician Galen in terms of his historical significance. As Needham and Lu explain, Zhang Ji's *Cold Damage Disorders* was one of the most important medical treatises in China after the *Inner Classic,* and more important than the *Inner Classic* from the perspective of drug therapy.[2] Since the eleventh century, this treatise has represented a key text in the classical medical tradition. Healers have read, memorized, and reflected upon the contents of the treatise, relying upon it for guidance in the diagnosis and treatment of ills.

At first glance, Zhang Ji would seem to be an odd choice of subject for my study, as one would not think that his image changed much over the centuries. If we turn to his preface to the *Cold Damage Disorders*, we find the image of Zhang Ji that dominates current accounts of the medical tradition. By Zhang Ji's account, the epidemic that struck the late Han dynasty (ca. 196–220) all but wiped out his clan – no less than two-thirds of his relatives succumbed to the epidemic in the space of a decade. Frustrated by his inability to rescue his kinsmen, or in his words, "moved by the fallen of the past and pained by those who could not be rescued from their untimely demise," the Han dynasty healer set his mind to rectifying the situation. "I have sought," he wrote, "the teachings of the ancients, selecting widely from the multitude of formulas." Not content with merely collating ancient works, Zhang Ji verified the efficacy of old formulas through his own trials. The result of his labor was a work called the *Cold Damage Disorders*, which explained how to diagnose and treat these illnesses. "Although this work cannot cure all illnesses," he remarked modestly. "I hope that readers will be able, when they examine a disorder, to recognize its source."[3]

The image of Zhang Ji as a tragic figure has captured the imagination of centuries of medical authors and healers. The early Qing scholar and authority, Cheng Yingmao 程應旄 (seventeenth century), for example, asserted that the preface to the *Cold Damage Disorders* was the key to unlocking the meaning of the treatise as a whole. As this seventeenth-century scholar put it, "When I read Zhang Ji's preface to the *Cold Damage Disorders*, I realized that it was precisely a work that 'lamented to Heaven and grieved for the people.'" Only by considering the preface, Cheng reasoned, would the reader see the parallels between the medical treatise and the *Spring and Autumn Annals* (*Chunqiu* 春秋), a classic long attributed to Confucius.[4] With this comparison, Cheng was alluding to Sima Qian's own preface to the *Records of the Grand Historian*, where the Grand Scribe of the Han had framed the act of writing as an expression of the sage's frustrations. According to Sima Qian, Confucius produced the *Spring and Autumn Annals* during a particularly difficult moment in the life of the sage. Unable to find employment as a minister, Confucius had failed to restore humane governance. As a result, Confucius had no choice but to encode his thoughts in his annals. Or, to quote Sima Qian, "Confucius transmitted the events of the past, thinking of those to come."[5] Cheng's comparison of the *Cold Damage Disorders* to the *Spring and Autumn Annals* is intriguing. For it suggests that Cheng saw Zhang Ji as a medical counterpart to Confucius, whom Cheng described as a sage and tragic figure.

The casting of Zhang Ji as a tragic figure captivated not only premodern scholars but also contemporary historians, who also believe that this figure is historical. Indeed, many modern accounts return to the preface in an effort to put the monumental treatise in its rightful historical context. In the *History of Chinese Medicine*, Li Jingwei 李經緯 opens his description of Zhang Ji with a bit of dramatic flair – by recounting how the great Zhang Ji emerged from the "turmoil" of late Han society, in the "unending flames of war," frequent ecological disasters, and last but not least, the terrible epidemic that wiped out Zhang Ji's clan. It was this epidemic, Li writes, that spurred Zhang Ji to devote himself to the study of medicine.[6] A similar image of Zhang Ji appears in *Traditional Chinese Medicine*, where Liao Yuqun reminds us that Zhang Ji's work on medicine was inspired by personal circumstances. "In AD 196 about two thirds of his family members died of cold disease," Liao comments, "and this tragedy inspired Zhang Zhongjing [i.e., Zhang Ji] to devote his life to the study of medicine."[7] Chinese scholars are not alone in locating the genesis of the *Cold Damage Disorders* in the healer's personal circumstances. Similar accounts of Zhang Ji's motives for studying medicine appear in a host of twentieth- and even twenty-first century presentations of the figure. Marta Hanson, for example, uses the preface to the *Cold Damage Disorders* to bring to life the world that gave rise to the treatise, connecting the events described in the preface to a well-documented epidemic that devastated the Han empire around AD 217.[8]

In part, the appeal of the preface can be well imagined. The preface seems to offer a tantalizing glimpse of an ancient healer speaking in his own voice, something rarely seen in other early sources. In this, the preface offers a contrast to the anonymous works discovered by archaeologists in tombs, generally understood to be the products of many hands. And in this respect, it stands even in relief to the biography of the Granary Master. Although Sima Qian narrated a large portion of the chapter through what sounds like the Granary Master's voice, one must remember that the Han figure never explained his motives for composing the document; the reasons were instead supplied by the scribe. With the preface to the *Cold Damage Disorders*, however, we see something different. Zhang Ji provided a personal narrative, explaining in his own words why he composed the *Cold Damage Disorders* – in other words, what set of circumstances prompted him to collect old formulas and to try them out.

Yet one should *not* assume that the preface preserves the voice of the historical Zhang Ji. The tragic persona found both in the preface and in modern histories emerged long after the Han dynasty. As we shall see in the following text, Zhang Ji's image, in fact, was kaleidoscopic; it changed as the contents of his corpus shifted in the process of transmission and editing over many centuries. His image moreover varied according to the preferences and goals of later interpreters.

To demonstrate Zhang Ji's kaleidoscopic quality, this chapter begins by tracing the representations of the Han dynasty healer over time. Through such methods, it demonstrates that one cannot find any trace of Zhang Ji's personal tragedy in editions of the *Cold Damage Disorders* or manuscripts dating before the eleventh century – *eight* centuries after his death. Instead, the familiar image of the man emerged belatedly – and due to interest in the figure's motives for writing his treatise. Such interest, furthermore, came out of the ranks of the Song and Yuan literati, who adopted healing as their métier in numbers for the first time. In order to present the arts of healing as a pursuit worthy of gentlemen, these healers transformed Zhang Ji into a sage by superimposing textual fragments over the image of Confucius. Zhang Ji's familiar image thus represents a *bricolage*, an artifact of medieval editors and healers who reshaped the archive according to their tastes.

SETTING THE STAGE

As our story moves well beyond the confines of late antiquity, it is worth clarifying what exactly it is that scholars refer to as China's medieval or middle period. By most accounts, antiquity in China ended with the collapse of the Han dynasty in AD 220 and the beginning of the Six Dynasties period (AD 220–589). During this era, China proper was ruled by a succession of competing houses in the north and south. This period of disunion only came to an end in the sixth century, with the founding of the brief Sui 隋 dynasty (AD 581–618), followed by the long-lived Tang (AD 618–907) and Song (AD 960–1279). Whereas the Sui and Tang ruled over vast empires that rivaled the Han in scope, the Northern Song hold of China proper proved more tenuous. Due to the rise of nomadic powers to the north and west, Song territory shrank greatly (see Figures 13 and 14). After a major defeat from one such power, the triumphant Jurchens, the Song court fled, moving its seat to the south in 1127. Meanwhile, the Jurchens established their Jin 金 dynasty (1115–1234) to the north, only to be conquered by the Mongol Yuan, with the Song falling less than fifty years later in 1279.

While historians generally agree as to when the medieval period began, less of a consensus exists as to when exactly it ended. Did medieval China end with the destruction of the Tang political order in 907, or rather with the fall of the Song dynasty in 1279? The lack of consensus sheds light on the fact that the term *medieval*, a category obviously borrowed from European historiography, fails to capture the dynamism of Song

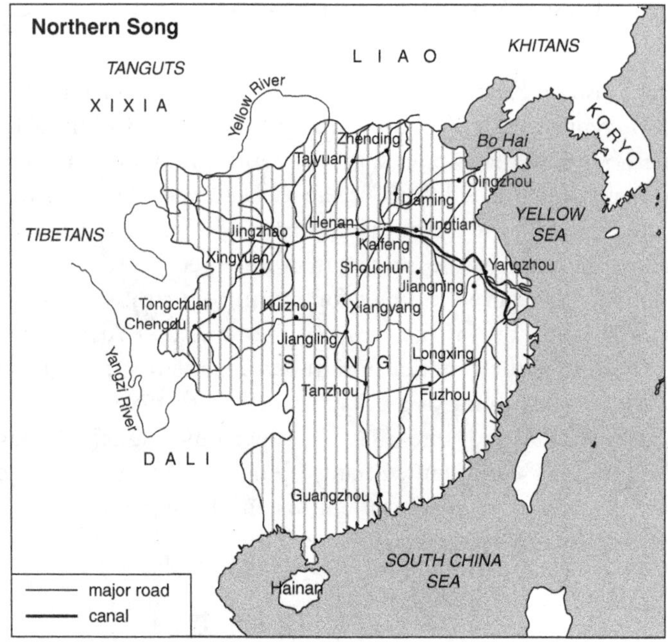

Figure 13 A map of the Northern Song, AD 960–1127.
Source: Patricia Ebrey, *The Cambridge Illustrated History of China, 2nd Edition* (2010), 137. Reprinted with permission from Cambridge University Press.

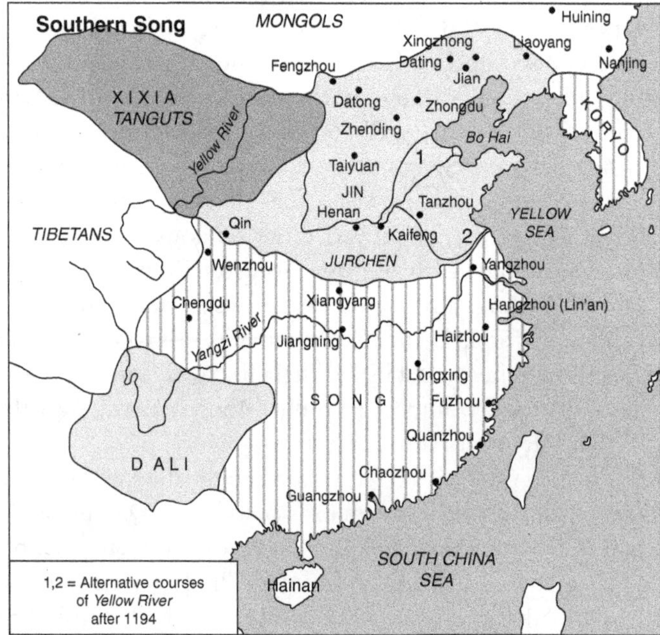

Figure 14 A map of the Southern Song Dynasty, AD 1127–1279.
Source: Patricia Ebrey, *The Cambridge Illustrated History of China, 2nd Edition* (2010), 137. Reprinted with permission from Cambridge University Press.

society. Pointing to the examination system and advanced bureaucracy, monetized economy, and print capitalism, scholars have made a persuasive case that the Song had many of the hallmarks of early modernity.[9]

It is the last of these developments, the emergence of print, that acquires special importance to our story. Regarded as the genius of the Song, print technology had matured in the middle of the tenth century. By most accounts, the development contributed to an upsurge in the printing of books, now cheaper and easier to produce than the handwritten manuscripts that they eventually supplanted. Such a development also allowed the Song court to take advantage of the new technology to sponsor the mass publications of various kinds of works.[10] These included medical treatises by the great luminaries of the Sui and Tang dynasties: the *Secret Essentials of the Outer Terrace* (*Waitai miyao* 外臺秘要; comp. eighth century) of Wang Tao 王燾; and the *Essential Prescriptions for Emergencies Worth a Thousand Gold* (*Beiji qianjin yaofang* 備急千金要方) and the *Supplemental Formulas Worth a Thousand Gold* (*Qianjin yifang* 千金翼方), both attributed to the great medical authority and healer, Sun Simiao 孙思邈 (581–682). The Song court also published a mass print edition of Zhang Ji's *Cold Damage Disorders*, from which current versions of the text derive.

Having established the historical context around Zhang Ji's life, I provide a précis of the preface. For the modern reader, the preface is a lurching philippic of thoughts and topics that do not seem to possess any commonalities. It opens with a tribute to Bian Que, "I am always moved to sigh with admiration," he wrote, "Each time I recall how Bian Que entered the state of Guo and examined the crown prince or how he determined the fact of illness merely by gazing from afar at the appearance of the Lord of Qi." The author then threw himself into a lengthy rant about the degenerate state of morals. "Men of the present," he thundered, "Compete for glory, standing on tiptoes around the powerful and influential, busying themselves in their midst. . . ." This pursuit of worldly things, the author further charged, caused them to neglect the art of medicine. Perhaps exhausted by his tirade, the author turned to the subject of his loss, recounting the epidemic that had killed two-thirds of his clan, his futile efforts to treat his kinsmen, and the methods he used to compose the *Cold Damage Disorders*. Without warning, the author then began a discussion of the *yin* and *yang*, and the Five Phases. Suddenly taken by yet another idea, his train of thought diverted to an introduction of the great exemplars of antiquity before enumerating the faults of healers in the degenerate present, their penchant for blindly following the traditions of their households, their shallow grasp of the classics, and their careless and perfunctory examinations of patients. And to all this, the author added a few more disingenuous comments about his modest abilities, bringing the text to its awkward close.[11]

As the overview indicates, the preface is a fascinating but ultimately disjointed document. Typical of works reconstructed from textual fragments, its helter-skelter quality leaves the reader to wonder what may have been lost, or better still, inadvertently added, in the process of transmission. More to the point, the preface's current state invites the reader to look more closely at the author's persona and to scrutinize its relationship to the historical man.

HISTORICAL PERSON OR MEDICAL PERSONA?

So what was the relationship between the present image of Zhang Ji and the historical man? To return to a question posed in earlier chapters, should one exploit the story about the epidemic for biographical data about the third-century personage, or should one think of it just as lore? To answer this question, I investigate Zhang Ji's image over the centuries, showing that the tragic face developed relatively late, as it is unattested in sources dating before the eleventh century. Prior to this time, Zhang Ji's image was different; most medieval authors presented him as a magical healer and master of drug formulary, whose curative and diagnostic powers rivaled those of legendary figures like Bian Que. Taken together, the evidence suggests that the Han healer's tragic image should be thought of as a persona shaped by the prerogatives of later scholars rather than a historical personage.

Naturally, some will ask whether it makes sense to think of Zhang Ji as a persona. There is little about contemporary descriptions of him that is suspicious. Unlike Bian Que, modern accounts do not mention any miraculous cures or supernatural qualities. Instead, the details in the biographical sketches of him transmitted through the centuries are plausible. Most historians' accounts of the healer make only three claims, none of which are outlandish in the slightest: namely, that Zhang's style name was Zhongjing 仲景, that he served as the governor in the southwest during the early third century, and that he composed the *Cold Damage Disorders*, which was subsequently edited by the court physician Wang Xi in the mid-third century.[12]

While all this would seem straightforward enough, scholars have contested the aforementioned facts for centuries. Take the issue of whether Zhang Ji had been an official. Premodern authors commonly referred to the healer as the Governor of Changsha or "Zhang of Changsha," a claim that at least one modern historian has disputed. True enough, a stele excavated in 1981, purporting to date from the early fourth century, mentioned a healer who had been the governor of the commandery. Even so, the existence of the stele does not prove that Zhang Ji had been an official. Based on its anachronistic language and the late style of its calligraphy, Li Jingwei concludes that the stele most likely postdated Zhang Ji's time by at least a millennium.[13] Sources closer to Zhang Ji's time, furthermore, never mentioned any governor of Changsha with the same name.[14]

Making matters worse, the current version of the preface probably took shape long after Zhang Ji's time. There are, in fact, signs that its contents, and in particular the story about the epidemic, resulted from centuries of textual accretion. As my arguments on this point are technical, even tedious, allow me to just summarize my findings in the following text (specialist readers are invited to read the appendix). My findings are as follows. By comparing surviving manuscripts and quotations in other sources, one finds that the contents of the preface changed over the centuries leading up to the eleventh century. At some point before that time, someone removed older contents, particularly descriptions of Zhang Ji's network of students and teachers, from a preface attributed to the Han healer. Later, probably in Tang, the editor or copier rearranged existing material, and also elevated portions of commentary into the main text. At the same time, someone else added new passages to the preface, including a passage recounting the story about the epidemic.

Besides questions about the dates of the current preface, there are other reasons to wonder whether the present image of Zhang Ji originated in the third century AD: early medieval sources offer no corroboration for the story that Zhang Ji wrote his treatise in the wake of an epidemic. The account from early medieval times most similar to this one is the *AB Classic* by Huangfu Mi. There, Huangfu Mi confirmed that the Han dynasty healer authored a treatise: "Zhang Ji expanded upon the decoctions discovered by the ancient sage minister Yi Yin, thus creating a work of ten rolls based on many of his own trials." Huangfu Mi furthermore remarked on Wang Xi's role in rearranging the *Cold Damage Disorders*, which he praised. "This arrangement of the text," Huangfu Mi commented, "was extremely concise, and the matters discussed there were practical."[15] Although Huangfu Mi attested to the fact that Zhang Ji composed a medical treatise, his remarks shed little light on the circumstances that spurred the earlier healer to compose his masterpiece. They also say nothing about any epidemic.

The absence of references to the epidemic in early medieval sources is telling because more than a hundred references to him survive in medical treatises, catalogues, anthologies, and encyclopedias written between the third and the eleventh centuries – in Huangfu Mi's preface to the *AB Classic* and his writings on drug formulary, the *Formulas for Emergencies Worth a Thousand Gold*, and the *Secrets of the Outer Terrace*, to name a few.[16] All this is surprising because the authors of these sources invoked Zhang Ji's memory, quoted from his corpus of works, and even praised him as the "progenitor of the myriad formulas."[17]

The silence around the epidemic is all the more surprising when one considers that medieval authors provided no shortage of details on Zhang Ji's life, career, and attitudes. Huangfu Mi, for example, talked about Zhang Ji at length in his various medical writings. Huangfu explicitly compared the earlier figure to other exemplary healers: "Bian Que and the Granary Master had nothing on Zhang Ji." At the same time, Huangfu Mi ranked Zhang Ji below Hua Tuo, one of Zhang's contemporaries. According to Huangfu Mi, Hua Tuo would treat his patients "by cutting through the belly and cleansing the five visceral systems."[18] Thus Huangfu Mi concluded, "Zhang Ji did not come up to Hua Tuo as a healer."[19] In this regard, Huangfu Mi was not alone. Authors writing before the eleventh century, in fact, discussed Zhang Ji avidly. These authors related his career as an official, and his meeting with the master healer Zhang Bozu 張伯祖, who predicted Zhang Ji's great potential. In addition, they described Zhang Ji's surgical prowess,[20] and enumerated the names, accomplishments, and works of Zhang Ji's pupils.[21] Such sources, which included manuscripts dating to Tang, even revealed the healer's polemical streak.[22]

Making matters worse, Zhang Ji assumed a different persona in medieval sources: there, he was not a tragic figure, frustrated by his inability to cure, but rather a magical healer with supernormal powers. To see this, let us turn to a story that circulated in the Six Dynasties and Tang eras, which was recounted first by Huangfu Mi. The story goes as follows: Zhang Ji once encountered a young official, who was still a lad. Zhang Ji had only to look upon the lad to know that something was terribly wrong. "You sir have an illness," Zhang Ji told the young man. "When you reach the age of forty, your eyebrows will fall out and within half a year of this, you will die." The illness, Zhang Ji added, was far from untreatable. "I would have you take the five-mineral decoction to prevent it," he said to the young man. Zhang Ji's warnings fell on deaf ears, however. Several days later, Zhang Ji asked the lad whether he had taken the medicine. Attempting to put the healer off, the lad answered that he had, but Zhang Ji was not fooled; a visual inspection confirmed that the lad had not complied with Zhang Ji's directions. Twenty years later, however, the eyebrows of the stubborn patient fell out as Zhang had predicted, and before the year's end, the patient was dead.[23]

It would be worth explaining how the story suggests Zhang Ji's evolving persona. In this connection, one must bear in mind that the Zhang Ji here offered a contrast to the tragic figure. The author who told the story about Zhang Ji depicted him as an extraordinarily prescient figure. Zhang espied the sprouts of illness not only before the afflicted experienced discomfort, but *decades* in advance. As readers will notice, this representation of Zhang Ji harkens back to the Bian Que from *Master Han Fei*. Like Bian Que, Zhang Ji appeared as a seer, capable of feats that surpassed the abilities of any normal healer. In this regard, nothing could be farther from the tragic figure found in the preface to the *Cold Damage Disorders* – a figure inspired to learn medicine precisely because of his inability to cure his relatives and who painstakingly collected old manuscripts before he was able to treat successfully, as he put it, *some* illnesses.

Indeed, we must wait many centuries before there are signs that medieval authors associated Zhang Ji with any epidemic or personal tragedy.[24] Recovered from a Japanese library, a manuscript version of the *Cold Damage Disorders* dating to around 1060 provides the first glimpse of the epidemic.[25] This manuscript is unique insofar as it contains large portions of the preface – something missing from earlier Tang manuscript versions of the text. A second reference to the epidemic appeared not long afterward: in the Song edition of Zhang's treatise published in 1065, a development discussed at length. Interestingly, the Song editors gave little attention to the story about the epidemic. Like earlier authors, these Song editors chose not to pronounce on the significance of Zhang Ji's brush with tragedy. Content with printing the preface in its entirety, they instead allowed readers to see for themselves the circumstances in which Zhang had written his monumental treatise.[26]

After the eleventh century, the story about the epidemic became prominent in discussions of Zhang Ji and his work.[27] In the *Supplements to the Lost Portions of Zhongjing's Cold Damage Disorders* (*Zhongjing Shanghan bu wang lun* 仲景傷寒補亡論), the important medical authority Guo Yong 郭雍 (1103–87) wrote, "Because in ancient times Zhang Ji had been 'moved by those who had fallen in the past and pained by those who could not be rescued from their untimely demise,' he composed the *Cold Damage Disorders*'; I, Yong have wholeheartedly sought to restore this work."[28] Another twelfth-century scholar, Yan Qizhi 嚴器之, framed the writing of the *Cold Damage Disorders* as a reflection of Zhang Ji's humaneness: "As to the disasters of the myriad illnesses, there is none so devastating as cold damage disorders." "Zhang Ji of Changsha," he added, "was thus 'moved by those who had been lost in the past and pained by those who could not be rescued from an untimely demise' and so composed the *Cold Damage Disorders,* comprising eleven rolls."[29]

The fact that this tragic face appealed to authors of the Song and Jin dynasties is evident even in works that told a slightly different version of events from the current preface. The important medical authority of the twelfth century, Liu Wansu 劉完素 (fl. 1186), also known as one of the Four Masters of Jin and Yuan, interpreted the remarks in the preface more liberally:

> 漢末之魏, 有南陽太守張機仲景, 恤於生民多被傷寒之疾, 損害横夭。因而輒考古經, 以述傷寒卒病方論一十六卷, 使後之學者, 有可依據。
>
> In the Wei at the end of Han, there was the governor of Nanyang, Zhang Ji, also called Zhongjing, who was moved by pity for the many people who suffered from cold damage disorders and who were stricken and died unnaturally. So, he examined all the old classics and on that basis wrote the *Treatise and Formulas for Cold Damage Disorders* in sixteen rolls, giving later students something to rely on.[30]

The passage presents several points of interest. For a start, the Song dynasty version of the preface said nothing about Zhang Ji's concern with the welfare of the population (and made no mention whatsoever of his tenure as the governor of Changsha). Instead, the focus remained on Zhang Ji's mourning for his lost kinsmen (*zongzu* 宗族). Although he evoked the wording of the preface, Liu's discussion represented a subtle reworking of the original themes. Note, for example, that Liu substituted the term *population* (*shengmin* 生民) for *kinsmen* in the current preface, thereby avoiding the suggestion that Zhang Ji was motivated by merely personal concerns. In so doing, he effectively cast Zhang Ji as an ancient sage who evinced an abiding love for all under Heaven.

The inconsistencies and gaps in the textual record cast doubts on whether the historical Zhang Ji created the tragic persona found in the preface. What is more, early medieval authors offered no corroboration for the tragic story about the healer. Not only did such authors pass over the episode in silence, but they also emphasized Zhang Ji's prowess as a magical healer. The familiar but tragic figure emerged only in the eleventh century. Though it made a belated appearance on the scene, this tragic persona soon eclipsed the earlier vision of the man as a supernormal healer. In sum, the evolution of Zhang Ji's persona suggests that medieval authors and healers had a hand in reshaping his image and the sources of his life long after his death.

MATTERS OF TIMING

Why did Zhang Ji's tragic face emerge so long after Huangfu Mi's time, namely, in the eleventh century? To answer this question, we will need to review two explanations, including the possibility that the changes in Zhang Ji's persona owed something to the rediscovery of the *Cold Damage Disorders* in the Song dynasty. After weighing the merits of this explanation, I then turn to a hypothesis that I favor: that framing Zhang Ji as a tragic sage and counterpart to Confucius reveals the emergence of a new kind of healer, literati who regarded medicine as an occupation. Such healers, I will further argue, cast Zhang Ji as a *sage* in an effort to win legitimacy. Such a move, in turn, necessitated new approaches to reading and interpreting the *Cold Damage Disorders,* approaches sensitive to the treatise's language and historical context.

Before turning to the hypothesis that I favor, I should consider a different explanation, one drawn from the recent literature. Might one attribute the fact that Zhang Ji's tragic face emerged belatedly to the rediscovery of his corpus in the eleventh century? In other words, perhaps early medieval authors did not mention the personal circumstances that inspired the treatise because the version containing the story about the epidemic did not come to light before the Song dynasty? This is a possibility suggested by the work of modern scholars such as Ma Jixing 馬繼興 and most recently Asaf Goldschmidt. Such scholars argue that the treatise only acquired canonical status when members of the Song Bureau of Medicine revised it and sponsored a small-character edition of the text for mass publication. Before that time, the text only circulated in fragments and in a very limited capacity, largely unknown to healers.[31]

Although Goldschmidt's findings have been subject to qualification,[32] the publication of the Song edition does explain in part why Zhang Ji's image underwent a makeover in the eleventh century. At the very least, the print edition made the materials in the current preface accessible to a broader readership, enhancing the chances that the story about the epidemic would be noticed by healers. Aside from this, the rediscovery thesis has an additional virtue, in that it accounts for the heterogeneous provenance and disjointed quality of the current preface, mentioned previously. In this regard, the testimonies of members of the Imperial Bureau of Medicine, who produced the Song edition of 1065, are key. When they set about the task of restoring the *Cold Damage Disorders*, the members of this bureau encountered a corpus in poor shape – or in their words, "riddled with errors, which had yet to be rectified." Making matters worse, the corpus was miscellaneous in origin, something obvious to the editors, who commented on the discrepancies in language.[33] And true enough, archaeological evidence reveals that the Song editors had been correct. The manuscripts discovered at the Dunhuang 敦煌 site reveal that medieval copiers commonly attributed apocryphal texts to Zhang Ji, for example, works that discussed personages who lived long after Zhang Ji's time.[34] Challenges notwithstanding, the Song editors did their best to make sense of the corpus. Working with earlier catalogues and attested parallels, they attempted to reconstruct the contents of the main text, the result being the *Cold Damage Disorders*, consigning the rest to the *Essential Summaries of the Golden Casket* (*Jinkui yaolüe* 金匱要略) and the *Classic of the Golden and Jade Casket* (*Jinkui yuhan* 金匱玉函).[35]

The theory that the print edition brought attention to Zhang Ji's new image has a final virtue; it explains the appeal that the story about the epidemic had for its Song dynasty audiences. According to Goldschmidt, the leading members of the Bureau of Medicine, such as Lin Yi 林億 (eleventh century), who were charged with editing the *Cold Damage Disorders*,[36] were largely concerned with the management of epidemics that plagued the Song empire. Indeed, the twenty years leading up to the publication of the print edition saw a sharp spike in epidemics.[37] These epidemics provided the editors with the impetus for restoring Zhang's treatises. The appeal of the tragic story for Song dynasty audiences can well be imagined, because Zhang's work paralleled the efforts of the government.

Still, the print edition of the *Cold Damage Disorders* cannot in itself explain the changes in Zhang Ji's image after the eleventh century. Even if one assumes that the restorative efforts of Lin Yi and the other Song editors made available obscure material, such an explanation falls short of accounting for the particular shape that Zhang Ji's image took after the eleventh century. This is because there were other possible ways of presenting the third-century healer. Another Song dynasty work, for example, recounted legends about the healer as an immortal, but such legends, interestingly enough, never became standard fare in Zhang Ji's hagiography.[38] Moreover, had the availability of the text been decisive, one would expect Zhang Ji's image to have changed overnight. But the Song editors of the treatise – the very men so concerned with the management of epidemics – failed to remark on the story found in the current preface.

In addition, the histories of medicine written in the following centuries – which provide synthetic and comprehensive accounts of Zhang Ji – passed over the epidemic in silence. These include the *Primer of Famous Healers through the Ages* (*Lidai mingyi mengqiu* 歷代名醫蒙求; thirteenth century) and *Discourses on Medicine* (*Yi shuo* 醫說; twelfth through thirteenth century). The authors of such texts presented Zhang Ji in the same way as earlier Tang dynasty works. Omitting all references to the tragedy, they instead recounted the outlines of Zhang Ji's official career. In addition, these authors also emphasized Zhang Ji's reputation as a supernormal healer, as someone who was the peer of Bian Que.[39] The descriptions of Zhang Ji were so close to Huangfu Mi's as to suggest that these authors had been influenced by that older presentation of the Han dynasty healer.

A fuller account of the shifting presentation of Zhang Ji requires considering an additional factor: the participation of the classically educated elite, or literati, in medical practice. As shown in the following text, such elites did not merely edit and publish mass print editions of the *Cold Damage Disorders*; crucially, they also designated its author as a sage, too. This designation, it will be further shown, reflected the fact that such literati healers framed medicine as a pursuit worthy of gentlemen and as a counterpart to the study of the ancient classics. For this reason, they read the *Cold Damage Disorders* as a classic, scrutinizing the textual remnants of antiquity in search of the hidden meanings of sages.

Before explaining how the literati reshaped Zhang Ji's image, it is worth saying a word about them. Such men, who referred to themselves as literati healers (*ruyi* 儒醫), took up the study and practice of medicine in several ways.[40] Like their Han and Tang predecessors, some of them wrote and edited treatises, including the statesman and literatus Su Shi 蘇軾 (1037–1101) and the high official and polymath Shen Kuo 沈括 (1031–95).[41] Such participation is also evident from the activities of the members of the Bureau of Medicine, who as Goldschmidt points out, were genteel men who practiced healing but *not* as an occupation.[42]

Beginning in the Song, some classically trained men – to be sure, a small minority of all healers – made their living from medicine.[43] This development represented a major break with earlier medical practice. In the Han, Six Dynasties, and Tang periods, it was common for members of the literate, office-holding elite to have authored medical treatises and to have tried their hand at the art of taking the pulse or making formulas, or even treating patients. Yet such men did not commonly stake their livelihood or main claim to fame on healing. After the Song dynasty, however, some literate men treated healing as their main occupation even though they counted among their friends, relatives, and patrons leading members of the literati and important officials. In this regard, another noted expert on the *Cold Damage Disorders*, Pang Anshi 龐安時 (1042–99), provides a prime example. The scion of a wealthy clan, Pang enjoyed the high regard of other literati because of his erudition. One of them, a famous poet, even graced Pang's work with a postface.[44]

Scholars explain the phenomenon of the classically trained healer, who practiced medicine as an *occupation*, in a variety of ways. Goldschmidt, for example, emphasizes the role played by imperial patronage. He argues that Song emperors took a particular interest in classical medicine and healing.[45] Some displayed their own therapeutic skills at court, while others compiled or sponsored formularies that bore their names. Others went so far as to write prefaces to important medical classics, asserting that healing was an endeavor worthy of rulers and gentlemen rather than a despised occupation.[46] Scholars such as Robert Hymes identify the importance of shifting household strategies in Song and particularly Yuan, strategies that encouraged wellborn and classically educated men to live by healing. This strategy reflected several interrelated factors: by Song times, the population had expanded but the size of the civil service had not, meaning that only a small handful of gentlemen would ever receive substantial rank within the bureaucracy.[47] The trend intensified in the Yuan dynasty, when the Mongols closed down the examination system for part of the dynasty and medicine enjoyed vigorous state support.[48] In response, elite lineages turned increasingly to healing as one of their next best options, citing the long-standing parallels between governance and medicine.[49] That medieval gentlemen saw healing as one alternative to official service was best summed up by a tenth-century minister, who worked on an imperial medical compilation: "In ancient times, if a sage did not reside at court," this minister observed, "He was invariably to be found in the midst of diviners and healers."[50]

Having discussed the potential reasons why literati adopted healing as an occupation, I turn to the effects of this development on the medical imagination, particularly the elevation of Zhang Ji as a sage in Song. All this differed greatly from the situation in Sui and Tang. Before Song, the *Cold Damage Disorders* did not have canonical status,[51] and authors did not refer to the third-century healer as a sage, a point made by Li Jingwei years ago.[52] The first surviving reference to Zhang Ji as a sage, in fact, appeared in the Song edition published by the Imperial Bureau of Medicine, a designation that apparently caught on. After the eleventh century, countless writers referred to the *Cold Damage Disorders* as a classic that expressed "the intent of a great sage."[53] Other authors demurred, instead awarding Zhang Ji the appellation of a second-class sage (*yasheng* 亞聖), a title used for Mencius.[54]

The reasons for Zhang Ji's elevation seem clear enough; he appealed to literati eager to demonstrate that healing was a genteel occupation.[55] For one thing, an early Song emperor had singled out Zhang Ji for praise, even going so far as to compare himself to the third-century healer.[56] The tragic face of Zhang Ji also happened to play well to the social conceits of elite healers. Seizing upon his reported place of origin in Nanyang 南陽 and the reference to a large clan, such healers took pains to demonstrate the connection between Zhang Ji and a powerful family of the same surname. In addition, such healers highlighted his official career, repeating the story found in the Tang dynasty *Record of Famous Healers* (*Mingyi lu* 名醫錄), where the author claimed that Zhang Ji had served a term as the governor of Changsha.[57] Given all this, it need not surprise that later commentators fused the story about the epidemic with reports of Zhang Ji's official career to claim that the Han figure, a virtuous official, had written the *Cold Damage Disorders* as an extension of his official duties. For them, Zhang Ji exemplified the complementarity of healing and governance. Just as the official treated the ills of the body politic, the elite healer tended to the woes of the body, thereby playing a part to ensure the health of the state.

Zhang Ji's designation as a sage transformed the way that scholars interpreted the *Cold Damage Disorders*, and it brought attention to the historical circumstances that produced the treatise. To see this, one must bear in mind that not all texts – or even ancient texts – merited the same kind of close scrutiny as classics in premodern China. The differences in attitude in part reflected assumptions about the gap between classics and more pedestrian forms of writing. Whereas works belonging to the latter class were assumed to be straightforward assertions, ancient and medieval readers treated classics as potent distillations of the Way. Hence, the frequent references to the abstruseness of the classics, and the necessity of "plumbing their subtleties" or "fully comprehending their mysteries." In concrete terms, this meant that scholars paid close attention to the language of ancient treatises, believing that the sage's message was encoded in the sequence and diction of the classic.[58] For all of these reasons, scholars vested great importance in understanding the historical moment in which the work was created, reasoning that the sage's form of expression reflected his circumstances. Take the famous example of the *Spring and Autumn Annals*, discussed in the introduction to this chapter. According to Sima Qian, a full grasp of this work required understanding that Confucius had been in a precarious position and had not been at liberty to discuss current events openly. When remarking upon ancient times, Sima Qian pointed out, the Master had used straightforward language, but when referring to sensitive matters close to his own day, the master was forced to employ an oblique idiom.[59]

The fact that healers saw the *Cold Damage Disorders* as a classic and the work of a sage is also apparent from remarks made by commentators. Unlike their predecessors, readers starting in the Song complained about the difficulty of grasping Zhang Ji's original meanings (*yiyi* 意義) and intent (*zhi* 旨) – that his meanings were hidden. As the members of the Song editorial bureau noted, "With respect to the work authored by Zhang Ji, its language is essential and mysterious and its methods are simple and clear."[60] In this regard, the members of the bureau were not alone. The aforementioned medical authority, Liu Wansu, described the *Cold Damage Disorders* as abstruse (*ao* 奧), an assessment consistent with the views offered by Yan Qizhi, Lü Fu 呂復 (fourteenth century), and others.[61]

The canonical status of the *Cold Damage Disorders* is finally apparent from the scrutiny that the text received from healers. Because classics were purportedly distillations of the Way, healers felt the need to examine the text closely to see whether it presented the actual utterances of the historical Zhang Ji, and to purge any interpolations and errors introduced by lesser men. In this respect, the attitudes of twelfth-century writers offered a contrast to earlier commentators. If such writers worried that Zhang Ji's message had been distorted through the process of transmission, they did not let on. Within a century of the publication of the Song print edition, however, scholars expressed concerns about the corruption of the sage's vision. One of the aforementioned Four Masters of Jin and Yuan, Liu Wansu, complained about editorial intervention. He charged that Wang Xi and other later commentators had polluted the "old teachings of Zhang Ji" with their personal perspectives. Writing of such commentators, Liu said, "They lost sight of the basic intent of Zhang Ji, and what they created was no longer consistent with the classic of the ancient sage, the result being that they added to the troubles of later men who studied the work."[62] Such a view of the treatise spread beyond the circles of healers and medical authors. A bibliographer of the Southern Song dynasty, Chen Zhensun 陳振孫 (fl. ca. 1211–49), similarly remarked that the language of the treatise was "laconic and archaic, as well as abstruse and refined."[63]

As we have seen, one cannot explain the changes in Zhang Ji's image by any single factor. For example, the mass publication of the *Cold Damage Disorders* does not in itself shed light on the pronounced interest in the treatise's origins, let alone the rising comparisons of Zhang Ji to Confucius. Instead, one must explain the prominence of Zhang Ji as a frustrated sage after the eleventh century by a confluence of factors. The literati's participation in the medical occupation did more than merely bring heightened attention to the treatise after centuries of neglect. More crucially, such a change introduced new ways of interpreting the work. Once readers saw the treatise as a classic, or a product of sagely genius, they focused on uncovering the author's intentions and thus became interested in its origins. All this opened the thinking of Song and Yuan healers to reenvision medicine as the complement to classical studies.

BEYOND SONG

One should *not* conflate the tragic figure of Zhang Ji – a fixture in modern historiography – with the historical man. The historical man is lost to us, and what we find in the textual record was a kaleidoscopic figure. In the Six Dynasties and Tang eras, he appeared as an authority on drug therapy and a magical healer, whereas in the Song and Yuan, he assumed a tragic persona, one modeled after Confucius, the sage *par excellence*. One may furthermore attribute such changes in Zhang Ji's image to several interrelated factors: the imperial publication project of the Song court, which brought to light the story about the epidemic; and the emergence of classically educated men who made healing their occupation and who used the story of the epidemic to frame Zhang Ji as a sage. Viewed from this perspective, one might say that the transformation of Zhang Ji into Confucius's medical counterpart owed much to the efforts of literati healers, who sought legitimacy for their craft by aligning it with the study of the classics and the art of governance.

The kaleidoscopic quality of Zhang Ji relates to the broader thesis of this book in several ways. To begin with, the case of the legendary healer shows that medieval editors and healers partook of the same model of cultural production as their ancient predecessors. Like Warring States and Han chroniclers, persuaders, and bibliographers, these medieval men were *bricoleurs*. Such men did not create the tragic image of Zhang Ji from scratch but instead worked with what was at hand. Like the preimperial chroniclers who fashioned the familiar images of Attendant He and Bian Que, medieval authors appropriated existing tropes to remake Zhang Ji according to their own preferences. And like Sima Qian, they also cut and pasted pieces of the preface, which had previously been formed into a tapestry tale out of textual remnants. By cobbling together disparate textual resources and pieces of legends, these medieval authors imbued older textual materials and Zhang Ji with new meanings and functions.

The case of Zhang Ji also reveals how the medical archive was shaped continuously by the work and agendas of premodern editors. These include the Song editors who transmitted, anthologized, edited, and published the critical editions historians still use today. Yet these Song editors were not alone in remaking the archive. In interpreting Zhang Ji's work, Song dynasty healers also had a hand in turning the kaleidoscope. By focusing on the story of the epidemic, they presented Zhang Ji as a sage and counterpart to Confucius, thereby bringing attention to the tragic image that continues to dominate presentations of the healer to this day.

It remains to say a word about whether Zhang Ji retained his kaleidoscopic quality in later periods of Chinese history. While a thorough answer to the question lies outside the scope of this chapter, there are signs that Zhang Ji's image, in fact, continued to evolve after the publication of the Song edition in 1065. As Marta Hanson shows, the fall of the Song witnessed the rise of new currents of medical learning in the teachings of Liu Wansu and the other masters of Jin and Yuan. For their part, such masters called into doubt the therapeutic relevance of the *Cold Damage Disorders* on the grounds that the illnesses of antiquity were dissimilar to those of their times, particularly those found in China's south. Such controversies, Hanson argues, in turn affected the way that later healers subsequently remembered Zhang Ji. For some medical authors, Zhang Ji remained an apical progenitor, "the ancestor of all formulas." Yet for others, Zhang was merely one of many sources of competing medical traditions.[64]

The challenge of the Four Masters was not the only sea change that occurred in medicine. The twentieth century also saw a wholesale attack on the classical medical tradition by modernizers and proponents of Western medicine. Despite such changes, Zhang Ji continued to command a prominent position in twentieth-century histories of medicine. Such a phenomenon raises a number of questions, including how the classical medical tradition managed to survive the attack. Did such attacks prompt a thorough remaking of this figure and other medical ancestors? And in an era committed to progress and the overhauling of Confucianism, how did the fathers of medicine fare? To answer these questions, the final chapter will consider the case of the last medical father, Huangfu Mi.

6

HUANGFU MI: FROM INNOVATOR TO TRANSMITTER

FOR OUR FINAL ACT, WE TURN TO A SEEMINGLY UNLIKELY choice of ancestor, Huangfu Mi. I say unlikely because at first glance, the third-century figure would seem to have little appeal as an ancestor. Huangfu Mi is not associated with any novel discoveries or miraculous cures. On the contrary, he suffered from congenital illness and spent most of his life in retirement in the provinces. Indeed, modern accounts do not leave the impression that the third-century man was even much of a healer. In his preface to the *AB Classic*, Huangfu Mi spoke of the extraordinary feats performed by Zhang Ji, but who were Huangfu Mi's patients? *Were* there even patients? In short, what moved Needham, Lu, and other historians to include Huangfu Mi among the fathers of medicine?

Primarily remembered as an editor, Huangfu Mi cuts an unglamorous figure in the tradition; scholars usually laud him for his meticulous editing rather than for any innovations or original treatises. Mansvelt Pokert, for example, says that Huangfu Mi, "revised the passages of the *Nei-ching* [i.e., the *Inner Classic*] dealing with sinarteriology, systematically filling out and redefining the terminology and the correspondences between foramina and symptoms."[1] Paul Unschuld, in turn, writes of the third-century man as the first editor and compiler of the canonical work. As Unschuld puts it, "Huangfu Mi did not add text himself; his objective was to present data he considered helpful in classical medicine."[2]

Such remarks epitomize the sentiments of twentieth-century scholars, particularly those writing in Chinese. For his part, Chen Bangxian (see Introduction) describes Huangfu Mi as an erudite man, who studied the classics while tilling the fields. After he became ill, Huangfu Mi purportedly turned to the study of medicine, acquiring a penetrating understanding of the classics and formulas. It was on this basis that Huangfu "authored the *AB Classic* and the *Classic of the Needle*, which circulated in the age."[3] Similarly, the authors of the modern primer, *Ancient Medical Texts* (*Yigu wen* 醫古文), refer to the *AB Classic*, the work that bears Huangfu Mi's name and largely defines his modern reputation, as "our nation's earliest treatise on acupuncture." According to these authors, the *AB Classic* derived from earlier texts, for Huangfu Mi merely "restored, summarized, and rearranged" older materials.[4]

Historian Liao Yuqun scarcely hides his dismay over Huangfu Mi's lackluster career. In *Traditional Chinese Medicine*, Liao devotes little space to Huangfu Mi and questions whether the third-century figure did much healing at all. He writes, "There are in fact no historical records of Huangfu Mi's clinical practice and patients." Huangfu Mi's great reputation, Liao adds, is "entirely based" on the *AB Classic*, a derivative work. Ironically, it is Liao Yuqun's unflattering depiction that makes the third-century figure look the most interesting. Unimpressed with the earlier figure, Liao Yuqun discusses Huangfu Mi's physical state of degeneration, a state that drove the third-century man to take a poisonous compound referred to as cold food powder (*hanshi san* 寒食散). Despite clear evidence that revealed the powder's dangers, Huangfu Mi failed to see the error of his ways and continued to take the drug.[5]

Huangfu Mi's reputation as an editor of ancient texts – or as the *Analects* might say, a transmitter rather than an innovator[6] – seems richly deserved. Even a cursory comparison of Huangfu Mi's treatise to surviving editions of the *Inner Classic* suggests that the third-century man had been a *bricoleur*. In composing the *AB Classic*, Huangfu pieced together parts of existing works, and he admitted as much: "I have compiled and collected writings on the three sections of the *Inner Classic*, thus making the things described and categories cohere with each other, omitted superfluous words, exorcised the redundant, and discussed the most potent and essential parts of the text so as to arrive at a work of twenty rolls."[7] In this regard, Huangfu Mi could not sound more like a caricature of the Chinese scholar. Here, he did not claim to add anything new to an existing body of knowledge. Instead, his contribution entailed filtering and purifying the records of antiquity: checking editions, excising redundancies, correcting infelicities of transmission, and bringing to the surface the underlying unity obscured by apparent inconsistencies. Such remarks underscore the fact that Huangfu Mi saw medical knowledge in regressive terms: knowledge about the body, he thought, had to be salvaged from the scattered textual remnants of antiquity. And for this reason, Huangfu Mi would seem to have nothing new to say.

Given all this, one is tempted to sum up Huangfu Mi's contribution to medicine with words like *pedantic* and *derivative* rather than *innovative, iconoclastic,* or *revolutionary*. While the casting of a medical ancestor as an unoriginal scholar seems predictable enough, I would argue that this way of portraying the man was hardly inevitable. Liao Yuqun's matter-of-fact discussion, which alludes to Huangfu's struggles with a poisonous but addictive powder, hints of a more compelling, alternative narrative. As an arresting chapter by literary scholar Dominik DeClercq reveals, the life of Huangfu Mi did not lack for interest, or for that matter, the stuff out of which myths were made. In fact, the biography in the *Jin History* (*Jinshu* 晉書; seventh century) – narrated largely in the first person – suggests no shortage of pathos: a man who turned away from a life of pleasure seeking and indolence after the intervention of a virtuous stepmother, only to be paralyzed with chronic illness in midlife. At one point, the illness was so severe that Huangfu Mi was driven to the brink of suicide, a point often breezed over by modern historians. What is more, Huangfu Mi was much more than an editor or commentator. He could *really* write. Like the other literati of his time, Huangfu Mi had a penchant for baring his breast to the world and lamenting his woes. His corpus moreover reflects a vivid imagination and a taste for melodrama. No alien to writing about the fantastic or strange, Huangfu Mi indulged in reciting the miraculous cures performed by great healers of earlier times, as well as recording the anomalies that portended the founding of new dynasties.[8]

This chapter investigates the making of Huangfu Mi's modern face. It asks how current historians have come to see Huangfu Mi as an editor, a transmitter rather than an innovator. By following this line of inquiry, this chapter advances our understanding of the medical archive in several ways. To begin with, it complements the findings of the last chapter by pointing to the role that medieval editors played in mediating the contemporary historian's access to the distant past. At the same time, the discussion departs from Chapter 5 insofar as it investigates whether medieval reorderings of the archive fixed the meanings of particular figures. By interrogating this problem, this chapter demonstrates that premodern editors and anthologists did shape the current archive with their cutting and pasting. But such editors did not *determine* subsequent interpretations of the past. As an examination of Huangfu Mi's alternative history reveals, the archive contained – and still contains – the seeds for another story about the man.

A survey of medieval sources shows how Huangfu Mi's image, like that of Zhang Ji, changed repeatedly over the centuries. In the first half of the medieval period, authors had yet to identify Huangfu Mi as the prosaic editor of the *AB Classic*. Instead, they focused on Huangfu Mi's connection to a controversial powder: they avidly discussed his misadventures with the drug, his personal observations of the drug's side effects, and his methods for treating the symptoms of drug poisoning – methods derived from Huangfu's personal experience rather than received wisdom. One may further explain the medieval fascination with Huangfu's experiments with cold food powder by the controversies that raged over the drug in the Six Dynasties and Tang. Beginning in the eleventh century, however, a new and rather staid image of Huangfu Mi replaced the older persona. From this time, medical anthologists overlooked Huangfu Mi's association with the drug, calling attention instead to his meticulous editing. This new image of Huangfu Mi was an artifact of controversy – but a different kind of controversy, a textual controversy. Scholars who defended the Yellow Emperor's authorship of the *Basic Questions* emphasized Huangfu Mi's testimonies and his work on editing the classical text. At the same time, they promoted the picture of him as a mere transmitter rather than an innovator, arguing that Huangfu had only edited the revelations of ancient sages. Although this characterization dominated subsequent representations of the figure, stories of Huangfu's struggles with cold food powder never disappeared entirely from the record. As our final analysis will reveal, such stories were rediscovered in the twentieth century and adapted to new uses.

SETTING THE STAGE

Thanks to a lengthy biography in the *Jin History*, one can establish Huangfu Mi's coordinates in space and time with some certainty. We know, for example, that Huangfu Mi was born around AD 215 and died in 282.[9] He thus lived through the fall of the Han; the establishment of the Wei 魏 dynasty in 220; and the coup d'état that ushered in the Jin 晉 (265–420), not to be confused with the Jurchen competitor state of the Song mentioned in Chapter 5. (For maps of Huangfu's eras, see Figures 15 and 16.) Huangfu Mi's biography sets forth the details of his whole life, beginning with a wild youth, the onset of chronic illness in midlife, his consistent refusals to take office, and the circumstances surrounding his death.

The Jin history reveals that in the eyes of his contemporaries, the third-century man was much more than a medical author. Hailing from an illustrious clan that had produced officials since the Han dynasty – his ancestors included high-ranking administrators, important generals,

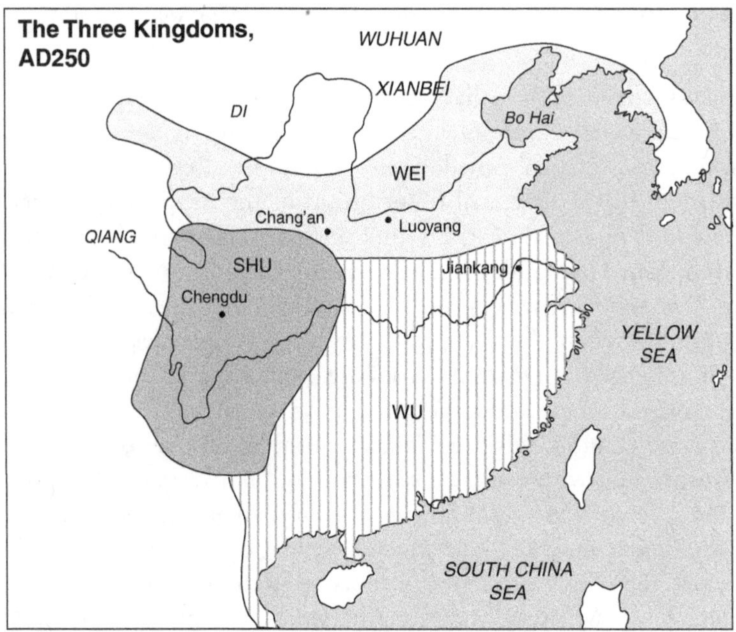

Figure 15 Map of the Three Kingdoms, ca. AD 250.

Source: Patricia Ebrey, *The Cambridge Illustrated History of China, 2nd Edition* (2010), 87. Reprinted with permission from Cambridge University Press.

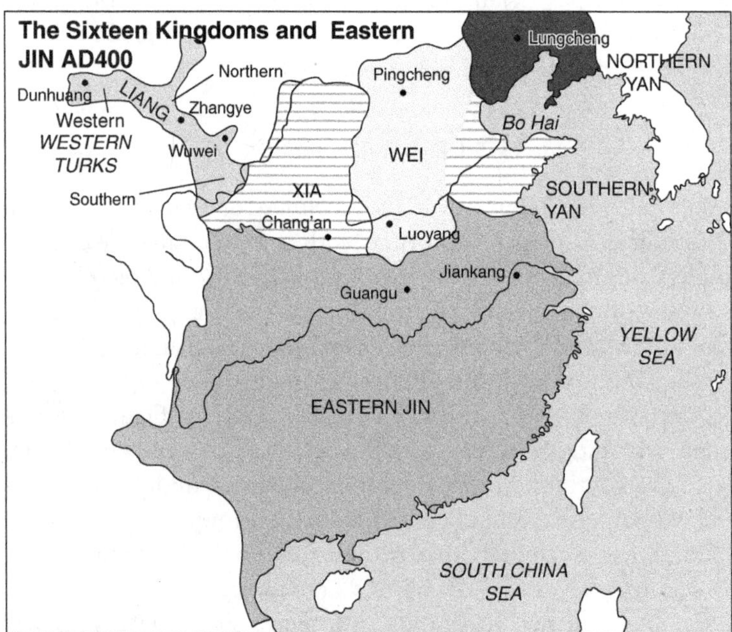

Figure 16 Map of the Sixteen Kingdoms and Jin dynasty, ca. AD 400.

Source: Patricia Ebrey, *The Cambridge Illustrated History of China, 2nd Edition* (2010), 87. Reprinted with permission from Cambridge University Press.

and respected classicists – Huangfu Mi stood at the top of the medieval social hierarchy.[10] Predictably, such a pedigree not only afforded him a splendid classical education but also made him a prime candidate for office.[11] Huangfu Mi also did his part in raising the prestige of his clan. Like the imperial bibliographer Liu Xiang, the third-century figure was a man of many talents, renowned for his breadth of knowledge. According to his biographer in the *Jin History*, Huangfu Mi wrote on a wide array of subjects and in different genres. He left behind a last will and testament, and wrote scores of highly regarded essays, memorials, histories, poems, autobiographies, and eulogies. He also collected anecdotes about lofty-minded gentlemen, recluses, and virtuous women for his compendia. Despite being concerned with subjects other than healing, two of these works, which bear on our discussion, require explanation. The first is the *Genealogical Records of Emperors and Kings* (*Diwang shiji* 帝王世紀), an influential work that traced the origins of the various ruling houses back to ancient sages. The second is "Rejecting Advice" (*Shiquan lun* 釋勸論), an essay that explored the question whether subjects (such as Huangfu Mi) were morally obligated to serve in office, particularly in cases in which the ruler was a tyrant.[12]

Besides these, a sizeable portion of Huangfu Mi's medical writings reaches the modern reader as compilations of different dates. Many of his ruminations on drug formulas – once set forth in titles such as the *Various Formulas Relied Upon by Huangfu Shi'an* (*Huangfu Shi'an yi zhufang zhuan* 皇甫士安依諸方撰) and a *Treatise on Cold Food Powder Formulas* (*Lun hanshisan fang* 論寒食散方) – now survive in large fragments within medieval compilations.[13] Such compilations include the *Treatise on the Origins of the Various Illnesses* (*Zhubing yuanhou lun* 諸病源候論) by Chao Yuanfang 巢元方 (fl. 605–616).[14] In addition, fragments of Huangfu Mi's corpus appear in a Japanese anthology, the *Essential Formulas of Medicine* (*Ishinpō* 醫心方) by Tanba Yasuyori 丹波康賴 (912–95).

Although it served as the basis of the imperial medical curriculum in the Tang dynasty,[15] the current version of Huangfu Mi's *AB Classic* is late; it derives from the eleventh-century edition published by the same members of the Imperial Bureau of Editing Texts that produced the mass print edition of the *Cold Damage Disorders*.[16] In terms of content, the *AB Classic* was a rearrangement of the materials found in two of the three current editions of the canonical *Inner Classic*: the *Basic Questions* and the *Classic of the Divine Pivot* (*Lingshu jing* 靈樞經).[17] The derivative quality of the *AB Classic* was something that Huangfu Mi acknowledged. In its preface, he explained that he collected and used materials from an existing work on acupuncture called the *Bright Hall* (*Mingtang* 明堂). As we shall see, this remark would acquire special significance in the eleventh century, when healers and scholars reimagined Huangfu Mi's contributions to the medical tradition.

Finally, a word about cold food powder, which I will reference repeatedly: the name of the drug is derived from its method of administration, as medieval elites often took the drug with cold food. The drug was also known by other names: the "five minerals" (*wushi* 五石), "rejuvenator" (*gengsheng* 更生), and "life preserver" (*huming* 護命). The name "five minerals" suggests that the drug was a mix of minerals – principals of Chinese pharmacopeia and mainstays in elixirs, including halloysite (*chishi zhi* 赤石脂), quartz (*baishi zhi* 白石脂/*baishi ying* 白石英), fluoritum (*zishi zhi* 紫石脂 / *zishi ying* 紫石英), stalactite (*zhongru shi* 鍾乳石), and sulfur (*liuhuang* 硫黄).[18] By Huangfu Mi's account, the drug appeared sometime in the Han dynasty and had even been used by the great Zhang Ji before falling into less able hands.[19] A libertine had discovered that the powder enhanced his sexual potency, and so the drug became popular overnight in the Han dynasty capital, with other wellborn men aping the practice. Making matters worse, the drug was soon used for all purposes: its potency relieved people who had long suffered from illness within the space of a couple days. Yet the powder also harbored hidden risks. As Huangfu Mi wrote, the common run of men "were overly fond of immediate gratification and oblivious to the calamities that would later befall them."[20]

WHERE DID THE TRANSMITTER GO?

Our sources and setting defined, we return to the central argument, that Huangfu Mi's portrait was hardly static through the ages, but bears the doctoring and decoupage of later scholars who retouched him to personify their own scholastic persuasions. Our survey of archival sources indicates that Huangfu Mi's medieval persona was very different from its present reincarnate. Authors before the eleventh century downplayed his exegetical work. Instead, they highlighted the figure's disastrous experiments with cold food powder. The interest in Huangfu Mi's misadventures with that medicament owed much to the controversies in medieval circles about the substance. Viewed from this perspective, the prominent association between Huangfu Mi and cold food powder reflected as much later medical debates about drugs as the man's self-fashioning.

Huangfu Mi was certainly a ubiquitous figure in the early medieval record – almost as ubiquitous, in fact, as Zhang Ji. Curiously, the first writers to mention the man said little about his editing. This is not to say that such writers were ignorant of Huangfu's interest in the curative arts, as such an interest was in fact noted early on. Take the annals written by a younger contemporary of Huangfu Mi, "[Huangfu Mi] was stricken by a wind that caused paralysis, and so he became knowledgeable about the classics and formulas."[21] Worth noting here is the fact that the chronicler made no mention of Huangfu's editorial work. In this regard, he was not alone; the catalogues of the Liang 梁 (502–557) and Sui dynasties mentioned Huangfu Mi's works on drug formulary but ignored his role in compiling the *AB Classic*.[22] What is more, they listed this last work without an author. Huangfu Mi's biographer in the *Jin History* was also silent about the man's efforts to edit older medical texts.[23]

The weakness of Huangfu Mi's connection to the *AB Classic* is surprising, particularly considering how often medical authors quoted from his corpus. Scores of references to Huangfu Mi survive in the vast medical compendia of the Sui and Tang dynasties. Yet, these only mentioned Huangfu Mi's name in connection to cold food powder. The *Origins of the Various Illnesses* provides one such example. Nowhere in this voluminous work did its compiler, Chao Yuanfang, relate Huangfu Mi's hand in compiling the *AB Classic*. Similarly, the Japanese compendium, the *Essentials of Medical Formulas*, referenced Huangfu Mi several dozen times – but once again, primarily in relation to drug formulary (we will discuss the one exception). The *Secrets of the Outer Terrace* of Wang Tao provides a different kind of example. Unlike other medieval authors, Wang quoted liberally from the *AB Classic* – all together more than a dozen times. Yet interestingly, the association with Huangfu Mi remained weak, as Wang linked Huangfu Mi's name to this text only once.[24]

Rather than presenting him as an editor of old works, medieval authors instead left the impression that Huangfu Mi's chief contribution lay elsewhere, in drug formulary and cold food powder. Such sources suggested a figure deeply knowledgeable about, if not obsessed by, that medicament. This is evident from the copious references to Huangfu Mi's explanations of cold food powder poisoning: the anguish, chills, fevers, pain, tenderness, insomnia, and suicidal thoughts that manifested the drug's deleterious effects.[25] In addition, the authors of such compendia related Huangfu Mi's admonitions about the drug, repeating his description of cases when men lost their lives or minds through careless administration of the substance: "Pei Xiu 裴秀 (224–271) of Hedong 河東 had taken the drug without moderation, and although he had the veneration of one who occupied the offices of the Three Excellencies, after he became deranged, he never regained his wits again."[26] Not content with citing just one of Huangfu Mi's remarks, the medieval editors also included the other cases of cold food powder poisoning described by the third-century man: "This is what had happened to my younger paternal cousin Changhu 長互, whose tongue shrank and entered his throat. Wang Liangfu 王良夫 of Donghai 東海 commandery suffered from an abscess that sunk into his back; the flesh along the spine of Xin Changxu 辛長緒 of Longxi 隴西 festered; and among my maternal cousins, six of them have died from the effects of cold food powder."[27]

The Huangfu Mi of medieval compendia also offers a contrast with the modern image in another respect: whereas modern scholars, especially Liao Yuqun, treat Huangfu Mi as an armchair physician, medieval authors presented the third-century figure as a highly effective healer. Indeed, the presentation of Huangfu Mi in these medieval compendia invites comparisons with Sima Qian's Granary Master (see Chapter 3). Like the Han healer, Huangfu Mi made no bones about announcing his track record of success with treating victims of cold food powder poisoning. Just as Sima Qian highlighted the Granary Master's successful prognoses, medieval editors displayed Huangfu Mi's boasts about his expertise. In addition, Huangfu Mi, who was something of a gossip, revealed the names of the patients he treated, calling attention to their prominent stations in life and the role that he played in their recovery. For example, he advertised his success in treating a governor, who had "sunken deep into an illness caused by cold food powder poisoning." Apparently, the governor was not alone in seeking Huangfu's help. Prior to that time, Huangfu Mi had used his drugs to stop another man's suffering and so that man recovered fully. As the healer explained somewhat immodestly, his efforts bore fruit; or in his own words, "from these cases, I became well known."[28]

Unlike modern descriptions of the man, which treat him as a transmitter of ancient wisdom, medieval sources depicted Huangfu Mi as an iconoclast – a figure whose knowledge of drug formulary stemmed not from ancient texts or authoritative figures but rather from the testimony of his eyes and ears. This is not to say that medieval authors thought of Huangfu Mi as an unlettered man, however. Through quotations, they showed him discussing different opinions regarding the origins of cold food powder, which he attributed to Zhang Ji. They provide a passage in which Huangfu Mi even explained the works that he consulted.[29] Oddly enough, Huangfu Mi gave earlier figures, including Zhang Ji, no credit for his treatment methods. On the contrary, Huangfu went to lengths to stress his own ingenuity. "All of these methods for saving the patient," he wrote, "have been things that I have personally experienced – having verified these methods through trial, I did *not* hear about them from anyone else."[30] More surprising still, Huangfu even asserted that his personal experience provided the source of his knowledge about healing: "It is only those who have 'broken their arm three times' [i.e., that are seasoned] that become healers, and it is not the case that one is born with knowledge, as trial and verifications are the sequence for learning."[31]

The medieval penchant for treating Huangfu Mi as an innovator is most obvious from the descriptions of the man's struggles with the drug. Sometime in his mid-thirties, Huangfu suffered from a debilitating bout of arthritis, an illness that would cause him to take cold food powder. As he explained it, the cure turned out to be worse than the actual illness. Unable to eat or drink and suffering from intense pain, Huangfu Mi was driven to the brink of suicide. By his own account, he grasped a knife with the intention of stabbing himself, only to be saved by members of the household who restrained him. After this close call, Huangfu took matters into his own hands. "I then withdrew," he told readers, "and reflected on the matter by myself." He then deduced that he would have to force himself to consume food and drink, and what was more, to plunge himself into *ice* water. By his account, this method, the hallmark of his treatment for cold food powder poisoning, proved effective. Huangfu's suffering thereupon came to an end.[32]

In large part, the strong association between Huangfu Mi and the powder reflected his self-presentation. Judging from what survives of his corpus, Huangfu wrote prolifically about cold food powder – and not merely in works concerned with drug formulary and medicine; the subject of his illness and cold food powder also consumed his writings on statecraft. Consider one of Huangfu's memorials, composed between 266 and 268, which dwelled on his misadventures with the mineral compound; an excerpt is translated in the following text based on Dominik DeClercq:

> 久嬰篤疾, 軀半不仁, 右腳偏小, 十有九載。又服寒食藥, 違錯節度, 辛苦荼毒, 于今七年。隆冬裸袒食冰, 當暑煩悶, 加以咳逆, 或若溫瘧, 或類傷寒, 浮氣流腫, 四肢酸重。於今困劣, 救命呼噏, 父兄見出, 妻息長訣。仰迫天威, 扶輿就道, 所苦加焉, 不任進路, 委身待罪, 伏枕 歎息。

> I have long suffered from a serious illness, which, for nineteen years now, has left half my body numb and my right foot smaller than the other. Moreover, I took cold food medicine for it but erred in the dosage, which caused me bitterness and acrimonious suffering, now seven years ago. In midwinter I stripped naked and ate ice, all the while feeling hot, vexed, and dejected. In addition, I was afflicted with coughs and reversal; at one moment I suffered from fevers and then chills, and at another, the illness belonged to the category of cold damage; the floating *qi* flowed down to swell my feet and my four limbs became sore and fatigued. At that point I was so debilitated that I could only save myself by swallowing and spitting – the family elders saw me and came outside, my wife and children bade farewell to me forever. I looked up to implore the majesty of Heaven, and supporting myself with difficulty, set out for the road which, however, only exacerbated the pain; it was beyond my strength to move forward and I gave up, waiting for the worst to happen. I leaned against my pillow and sighed.[33]

The passage, which describes the circumstances that drove Huangfu Mi to administer cold food powder, bears explanation. As DeClercq points out, Huangfu Mi wrote about his physical suffering on the occasion of declining official summons. The Jin court had just experienced a coup d'état. As the new ruler was eager to bolster his legitimacy by surrounding himself with men of renown, he naturally summoned Huangfu Mi, a leading luminary of the age and the scion of a great clan.[34] Huangfu Mi thus found himself in a quandary. He realized that working for this new tyrant could be fatal if the regime was short lived, because he ran the risk of being executed as a traitor. Snubbing the new ruler, however, was also a bad option, as it might incur equally dire consequences. The best out for Huangfu was thus to plead fragility due to sickness, and he did – with considerable panache.

Motives notwithstanding, the reasons why Huangfu Mi's misadventures with the powder came to dominate later representations are clear. The story – rendered in Huangfu's beautiful prose – supplied a vivid account of the ravages of illness. No other early figure in the classical medical tradition, in fact, claimed such a dismal failure of treatment. The story was thus both distinctive and memorable. All this is important when one considers the role of memory in early and medieval China. In such eras, readers did not only write, copy, and read stories quietly, but more often than not, they also intoned and delivered them orally.[35] The more distinctive the tale, the better the chances that it would capture the imaginations of its audiences and be preserved. Huangfu Mi's account of his illness moreover found its way into a highly visible source, his biography in the official history, or the standard reference for his life and works. All of this, in turn, further reinforced Huangfu's association with the powder.

One can also account for his association with the powder in terms of the medieval fascination with the substance. While scholars sometimes regard the powder merely as a third-century fad, members of the medieval elite, in fact, continuously ingested, discussed, and debated the powder seven centuries after Huangfu Mi's day.[36]

In addition, the controversies surrounding cold food powder – its origins, proper application, and, above all, its safety – also deepened the association between Huangfu Mi and the compound. Opponents of the powder asserted that the substance was too dangerous to be taken under almost any circumstances, citing the many adverse effects associated with it. The great Tang medical authority, Sun Simiao, for example, characterized the powder as nothing less than a "fearsome poison." Sun also attributed the popularity of the drug to the lechery of his contemporaries: "There are also those with an insatiable desire to eat the five minerals [i.e., cold food powder] due to seeking the pleasures of the bedchamber."[37]

In contrast, defenders of cold food powder went to lengths to minimize the pitfalls of the drug. Such defenders instead highlighted the virtues of the medicament. Wrote one author, "The powder is good for extending the lifespan and nourishing the vitality; it also harmonizes the nature and principle."[38] Although such defenders emphasized the potential virtues of the drug, they also acknowledged the risks involved in administering it. In this connection, one defender asserted that the compound was too tricky for mediocre healers, or those of "middling ability," to handle.[39] "Fatalities reflect mistakes in administering the drug," one said, "so the fault does *not* lie with the powder."[40]

Interestingly, it was the proponents of cold food powder who found the testimonies of Huangfu Mi to be of the greatest use. Such proponents marshaled the man's testimonies, particularly when arguing that fatalities reflected errors in administration rather than the intrinsic properties of the drug. They highlighted Huangfu's admonitions against using the drug casually or, as many did, with reckless abandon. In this connection, one proponent even singled out Huangfu Mi for praise as a "fine talent," while noting that his views about the proper uses of the powder were at odds with another authority. Whereas the third-century man had deemed it appropriate to cool the body, the author noted, others had urged patients to do the opposite and to apply heat. For such an author, the differences in opinion underscored the fact that the drug should only be taken by someone with a thorough understanding of the drug's intricacies.[41]

Medieval sources thus offer a different picture of Huangfu Mi than the one found in modern histories. Whereas modern historians remember the third-century figure primarily as an editor, medieval writers often depicted him as a victim of cold food powder poisoning, an effective healer, and an innovator. One might even argue that this medieval image of Huangfu Mi largely reflected later controversies about the powder. In such debates, Huangfu Mi's testimonies became a central rallying point, as defenders used him to argue that the powder was not inherently deadly, and killed only men who did not understand the drug. For them, Huangfu's experiences exemplified the trickiness of administering the drug, which defenders emphasized should be used only by the most skillful of healers. Given that medieval elites debated the virtues and risks of the powder, it need not surprise us that it was the image of Huangfu Mi plunging into ice baths that caught the attention of audiences.

THE EMERGENCE OF THE PEDANT

We have seen Huangfu Mi's other face, but when did the man's image begin to change into that of the pedant – and, more importantly, *why* did it change? In other words, how does one account for the prosaic image of the classical scholar eclipsing the more arresting vision of a sick man, experimenting with a potent but dangerous cure? To answer these questions, one must first establish when this shift occurred. As I shall demonstrate, this new image of Huangfu Mi became prominent after the mid-eleventh century, following the publication of the *AB Classic's* print edition. Such a shift, I propose, is best explained by the controversy that raged over the *Basic Questions* – a controversy that not only brought heightened attention to Huangfu Mi's efforts to compile the *AB Classic* (a mere "edition" of the *Basic Questions*), but also necessitated his transformation from an innovator into a transmitter.

Eighth-century authors were the first to refer to Huangfu Mi as an editor. One scholar, Yang Xuancao 楊元操 (sixth through seventh century), described the *Bright Hall*, one of Huangfu Mi's sources for his acupuncture treatise, as the "orthodox classic" of the Yellow Emperor. Yang also paid homage to Huangfu Mi's exegetical prowess, writing that the third-century figure had been a "great talent of the Jin court, who possessed a penetrating knowledge of the medical arts." By Yang's account, Huangfu Mi had used this wealth of knowledge to "compile the *AB Classic*, thereby setting forth the three parts [i.e., of the *Inner Classic*]."[42] Although it anticipated later treatments of the figure, Yang's characterization of Huangfu Mi was not influential, at least not overnight. Repeated only a handful of times over the next few centuries, such a characterization did little to alter Huangfu Mi's image as a proponent of cold food powder.[43] Instead, the connections between Huangfu Mi and the *AB Classic* only became pronounced in late Tang. The authors of the catalogues in the *Old Tang History* (*Jiu Tangshu* 舊唐書; 945) and *New Tang History* (*Xin Tangshu* 新唐書; 1060) corroborated the observations of Yang. They listed Huangfu Mi as the compiler of a text called the *Yellow Emperor's Classic of Acupuncture in Three Parts* (*Huangdi sanbu zhenjing* 黃帝三部鍼經), which was another name for the *AB Classic*.[44]

One must wait until the eleventh century, however, before we find clear signs that medieval authors preferred to present Huangfu Mi as an editor.[45] The preference for this image is on full display in the Song postface to the *AB Classic*, which the members of the Imperial Bureau of Medicine wrote in 1069.[46] Such bureau members described the third-century figure accordingly:

> 晉皇甫謐　。博綜典籍。百家之言。沉靜寡欲。　有高尚之志。得風痺。因而學醫。習覽經方。遂臻至妙。取黃帝素問、鍼經、明堂三部之書。撰為鍼灸經十二卷。
>
> Huangfu Mi of the Jin was broadly learned in the canonical works and the words of the hundred masters. He was deeply quiescent, had few desires, and possessed lofty goals. Because he fell ill with a paralyzing wind, Huangfu Mi took up the study of medicine, reading and becoming familiar with the classics and formulas. He subsequently arrived at their supreme subtlety. He took three texts, the *Basic Questions of the Yellow Emperor*, the *Classic of Needling*, and the *Bright Hall*, and edited them into the *Classic of Needling and Moxibustion* of twelve rolls.[47]

Although they depicted Huangfu Mi's brush with illness as his motivation for studying the healing arts, the bureau members omitted his misadventures with cold food powder. Instead, they focused on his editing of ancient medical works and his knowledge of the classics. While one might be tempted to chalk up their silence about cold food powder to ignorance, the evidence suggests the contrary. The bureau members also published a definitive edition of the *Treatises on the Origins of the*

Various Illnesses – the medical compendia that devoted so much space to Huangfu Mi's writings on the powder.[48] Their silence, in other words, reflected choice.

The presentation of Huangfu Mi as an editor has been undeniably influential. In later periods of Chinese history, authors seemed to be less taken with Huangfu's association with cold food powder than with his contributions in the *AB Classic*. In the *Discourses on Medicine* (twelfth through thirteenth century), Huangfu Mi appeared as a classical scholar who transmitted the learning of the Yellow Emperor and compiled his revelations into the *AB Classic*, rather than a man with an addiction.[49] The author never actually mentions Huangfu Mi's extensive writings on cold food powder, despite devoting a section to the medicament.[50] Similarly, the *Great Compendium of the Ancient and Modern Medical Tradition* (*Gujin yitong daquan* 古今醫統大全; sixteenth century) treated the *AB Classic* as Huangfu Mi's main achievement; quoting verbatim the descriptions in the Song edition of the *AB Classic*.[51] The depiction of the third-century man in the *Complete Records of Medicine* (*Yibu quanlu* 醫部全錄; seventeenth century), an anthology that drew upon a variety of earlier sources, is even more telling. The anthologist explained Huangfu's decision to study medicine as a response to illness, "Huangfu Mi studied the primary and secondary analyses so as to relieve the distress of illness." He also downplayed Huangfu Mi's connection to cold food powder, eulogizing instead his contributions to the *AB Classic*. Still, the author clearly made use of Huangfu Mi's biography in the *Jin History*, a source that detailed the symptoms the man suffered as a result of ingesting the powder.[52]

So how do we explain the fact that authors after the eleventh century remembered Huangfu Mi largely for the *AB Classic*? In this connection, allow me to begin with a disquieting possibility, one hard to ignore in light of my findings for Chapter 5 – to wit, the story of Huangfu Mi compiling the *AB Classic* is spurious. Perhaps we do not hear of Huangfu Mi's editing of ancient medical texts before the eighth century because he did no such thing? Adding to our suspicions is the fact that no trace of the preface survives in works predating the mid-eleventh century. As a result, one wonders whether the preface, the only definitive link between the *AB Classic* and the third-century figure, might have been the creation of Song editors, who exercised a considerable amount of creative license when editing the work.

While worth taking seriously, this possibility is not the best explanation of the change in Huangfu Mi's image in the Song dynasty. To begin with, the fact that the Liang and Sui catalogues did not list Huangfu

Mi as the compiler of the *AB Classic* is unsurprising; the names of editors were often omitted from medieval catalogues.[53] More importantly, Huangfu Mi's other writings support his authorship of the preface to the *AB Classic*. Take Huangfu Mi's famous claim that the Yellow Emperor and other ancient sages composed the *Basic Questions*. This, Huangfu Mi asserted not once but thrice – in two other works, the *Genealogical Records* and "Rejecting Advice" as well as the *AB Classic*.[54] In "Rejecting Advice," he even recited the history of the curative arts:

若黃帝創制於九經	Yes, the Yellow Emperor created the Nine Classics.
岐伯剖腹以蠲腸	And Qibo cut through the abdomen to cleanse the intestines.
扁鵲造虢而尸起	Bian Que went to Guo and revived a corpse.
文摯徇命於齊王	Wen Zhi sacrificed his life for the King of Qi.
醫和顯術於秦晉	Attendant He manifested his arts in the states of Qin and Jin.
倉公發祕於漢皇	The Granary Master expounded on his secrets for the Han sovereign.
華佗存精於獨識	Hua Tuo preserved his essence with techniques known only to him.
仲景垂妙於定方	Zhongjing [i.e., Zhang Ji] bequeathed the mysteries of medicine in his set formulas.
徒恨生不逢乎若人	I only regret that in this life I will not meet men such as these.[55]

The recitation should look familiar. There is the same historical progression that appears in the *AB Classic*; Huangfu began here with the ancient sages of high antiquity before moving through successive stages of the past down to the present. Likewise, many of the figures were the same, with minor variation (Huangfu substituted the legendary minister Wen Zhi 文摯, who cured his lord by infuriating him, for another figure of comparable status, Yi Yin). Such differences aside, readers familiar with the *AB Classic* will recognize many of the same names: the Yellow Emperor, Attendant He, Bian Que, the Granary Master, Hua Tuo, and Zhang Ji.

To explain the changing representations of Huangfu Mi, we are instead better served by looking at the shifting priorities of healers and medical authors. In part, the surge of interest in Huangfu Mi's exegetical contributions undoubtedly reflected the declining popularity of cold food powder. Although it never disappeared entirely from the Chinese pharmacopeia, the popularity of the powder waned in Song times.[56]

Consequently, one would expect that healers would have had to associate Huangfu Mi with other achievements; otherwise he would have faded from the history of medicine entirely.

Perhaps the single most important factor that explains Huangfu Mi's changing face was the controversy over the *Basic Questions*. As we will see, scholars from the Song dynasty began to emphasize Huangfu Mi's editorial skills precisely at the moment in which the authenticity of the *Basic Questions* was seriously called into doubt. For defenders of the *Basic Questions*, it became critical that Huangfu Mi appear as a transmitter, the preserver of ancient revelations rather than an innovator – or worst still, a clever forger.

Before explaining how such a controversy was responsible for the shifting presentation of Huangfu Mi, I must provide some background. Although not new, doubts about the provenance of the *Basic Questions* were especially pronounced in the eleventh century, when important scholars and officials questioned the Yellow Emperor's authorship of the classic.[57] Such men included a long list of scholarly luminaries. One of the most influential minds of the eleventh century, statesman and literatus Cheng Yi 程頤 (1033–1107), for example, openly voiced his doubts about the provenance of the *Basic Questions*, arguing that it was written at the end of the Warring States.[58] Such skepticism was shared by others, including Sima Guang 司馬光 (1019–86), another great eleventh-century statesman and literatus.[59] For his part, Sima Guang paid his compliments to the learning presented in the *Basic Questions*. But when asked if the text was the work of the Yellow Emperor, he rejected the possibility out of hand. "When the Yellow Emperor was governing the realm," he wrote, "he was in the Bright Hall busy receiving commands all day, and so how could he be discussing medicaments and needles with Qibo?" The *Basic Questions*, Sima Guang added, must have been the work of men of the Warring States or Qin, who assumed the name of the Yellow Emperor in order to win credibility.[60]

To see how the controversy over the *Basic Questions* affected Huangfu Mi's image, we should go to the postface of the Song edition of the *AB Classic*. Interestingly enough, the Song bureau members said little about the *AB Classic* in the postface, choosing instead to emphasize that the *Basic Questions* was the work of ancient sages. "There have been some," the bureau members complained, "who say that the three parts of the *Inner Classic* – the *Basic Questions*, the *Classic of Needling*, and the *Bright Hall* – are *not* the writings of the Yellow Emperor."[61] Readers familiar with the conventions of the era will notice the omission of names – specifically, those of Cheng Yi and Sima Guang. Such an omission must have been deliberate. Mentioning that the greatest minds and most famous officials of the age thought differently would not have helped the bureau members! Instead, they focused on the one literatus who agreed with them, Huangfu Mi. In many ways, the bureau members' choice to home in on Huangfu Mi made sense. To begin with, it was in the *AB Classic* that Huangfu Mi expressed his belief that the Yellow Emperor had written the *Basic Questions* and other important works. And Huangfu Mi furthermore claimed in the preface to have been nothing more than an editor, who collected and rearranged the revelations of the ancient sages.[62] What is more, the third-century man had a sterling reputation as a great scholar of antiquity, which undoubtedly lent cachet to the bureau members' argument. As they reminded their readers, "None of the ancient classicists over the ages have come up to Huangfu Mi."[63]

In this regard, the Song bureau members were not alone. One finds similar appeals to Huangfu Mi's authority in the *Discourses on Medicine*, where the author summoned Huangfu's testimonies when making a case for the ancient provenance of the *Basic Questions*.[64] Other defenders used Huangfu Mi in a more subtle fashion, while acknowledging the arguments of the opposition. For example, Lü Fu, discussed briefly in Chapter 5, not only acknowledged that the text was the product of disparate hands, but also of different eras. Lü even went so far as pointing out parts of the *Basic Questions* that were spurious – forgeries interpolated into the main text by a deceitful Tang commentator. Yet to his mind, such insertions did not detract from the importance of the work, as the *Basic Questions* still preserved the revelations of the ancient sages. In this regard, Lü noted, the medical canon was like one of the ritual classics, which had only taken its present form in the Han dynasty. Nevertheless, the text preserved the teachings of earlier ages, for it transmitted the wisdom of Confucius. According to Lü, the case of the *Basic Questions* was no different, as Huangfu Mi and later scholars had merely rearranged older materials that expressed the sages' subtle understandings of the body: the workings of the *yin* and *yang*, the Five Phases, the location of the acupoints, and so forth. Although Lü Fu's argument was far more sophisticated than those of the Song bureau members, there were certain commonalities. Lü also shared the Song bureau members' view of Huangfu Mi as a transmitter and editor, a status that set Huangfu Mi apart from other scholars. Whereas Lü branded one Tang commentator as a forger for adding new material into the *Basic Questions*, he saw Huangfu Mi as the faithful custodian of the sage's legacies.[65]

Our discussion thus suggests that the present image of Huangfu Mi evolved over time. Whereas in the Six Dynasties, Sui, and Tang, Huangfu Mi was seen as an effective healer, famed for his innovations in treating cold food powder poisoning; by the eleventh century, Huangfu had acquired the more prosaic image of an editor. One may furthermore explain this change by a host of factors, the most important being the debates about the *Basic Questions*. In such debates, the defenders of the Yellow Emperor's authorship marshaled Huangfu Mi's testimonies in their favor. In addition, Huangfu Mi's reputation as a classical scholar and transmitter played a critical role in arguments concerning the ancient origins of the medical canon. In an era when critics were quick to accuse others of surreptitiously introducing new content under the guise of preserving or discovering the lost revelations of antiquity, the fact that Huangfu Mi had nothing "new" to say proved to be a virtue.

CONCLUSION AND DISCUSSION

T. S. Eliot's phrase "Time future contained in time past" arguably captures our findings. As seen, attempts to retrieve the historical Huangfu Mi are as futile as ones to locate the real Zhang Ji. Like Zhang Ji, Huangfu Mi's image was kaleidoscopic; his characteristics changed depending on the perspectives and rhetorical aims of later interpreters. In the Six Dynasties and Tang periods, Huangfu Mi was synonymous with cold food powder, the drug that enjoyed great popularity and notoriety among the ruling elite of the medieval period. As a result, he assumed an important position in medieval debates about the powder. For defenders, Huangfu Mi's personal history, or better still, his moving performance as a sick man, embodied the risks of the drug – a drug, they insisted, that could only be administered with the utmost care. Beginning in the eleventh century, however, another more pedantic image of Huangfu Mi sprung to the fore. This shift reflected the emergence of another controversy, one revolving around the provenance of the *Basic Questions*. Defenders of the Yellow Emperor's authorship of the *Basic Questions* appealed to Huangfu Mi's testimonies in the *AB Classic*. Accordingly, they summoned Huangfu Mi's authority as a scholar and emphasized his editorial skills over his innovations.

Where does the case of Huangfu Mi fit within the larger arc of our argument? In part, the posthumous fate of the third-century figure is consistent with those of earlier medical fathers. As discussed previously, earlier figures, particularly Bian Que, were more legendary than historical and naturally lent themselves to being remade to match the storyteller's aims. At first glance, then, Huangfu Mi would seem to be too real to be malleable; the facts of his life, one would think, possessed a stubborn historicity that defied easy remolding. Despite what one might expect, Huangfu's historicity presented no obstacle to later *bricoleurs*, even ones with rigorous philological training. Without succumbing to outright forgery, the later *bricoleurs* found ways to adjust the narratives of Chinese medical history. Just as Han dynasty writers lifted rhetorical devices out of their original contexts, imbuing them with a new literal sense, these Tang and Song authors also pulled pieces of textual matter from earlier writings, mixing and matching their sources to create novel narratives about their ancestors. Alternatively, they focused on particular materials – homing in on specific texts, passages, and events. Through such a narrowing of perspective, these medieval authors recreated the image of the ancestor in ways that were congenial to them. Hence, one might say that the traces of the Tang and Song future can be glimpsed in the archives of the early medieval past.

Yet the scholars of the Tang and Song dynasties were not the only *bricoleurs*. The habit of recycling and reworking earlier resources – even while remaining faithful to established chronologies – survived into the twentieth century. The malleability of Huangfu Mi's persona is perhaps clearest in an account by Yu Jiaxi 余嘉錫 (1884–1955), a towering figure in twentieth-century historiography. Best known for the *Extensive Examples from Ancient Books* (*Gushu tongli* 古書通例), Yu is still touted by scholars as one of the best examples of the Doubting Antiquity movement. Like other members of this movement, Yu brought to his examination of China's historical record a rigorous and self-reflexive eye. Not content with merely dividing his sources between the spurious and authentic, Yu Jiaxi queried the very categories of historical analysis, questioning when notions of authenticity and authorship came into being. More strikingly, he sought to illuminate the social relations and practices of reading that authorized different modes of textual production and concepts of historicity. Aside from such endeavors, Yu Jiaxi also wrote a long essay about cold food powder. As one would expect, the essay bore testimony to Yu Jiaxi's massive erudition, for he brought to his analysis an impressive array of sources, which he dissected with his usual brilliance.

Most revealing in Yu Jiaxi's essay, however, is his treatment of Huangfu Mi, who is cited liberally. Curiously, Yu Jiaxi's discussion omitted any reference to Huangfu Mi's editorial activities, activities that the historian must have been aware of. In a move reminiscent of Tang medical thinkers, this modern scholar presented Huangfu Mi as the foremost expert of cold food powder, a prophet ahead of his own time. The reasons why Yu preferred the older Huangfu Mi are easy to guess. The essay was published in 1938, at the start of the second Sino-Japanese war, a period of social upheaval and Chinese military inferiority. For Yu Jiaxi and other members of the educated elite, China's opium epidemic was symptomatic of its weakness. In his own essay on cold food powder, Yu lamented the destructive power of opium, which he blamed for the decline in China's fortunes. How could something so bad for the health of the body, he mused, be so pervasive? In an effort to answer this question, Yu turned to the case of cold food powder, a malaise of an earlier age, which served as "warning to those who ingest and take pleasure in opium."[66] Much like his Tang and Song predecessors before him, Yu Jiaxi made his case by channeling the voices of antiquity. And for this reason, Huangfu Mi was called upon once more to don the role of the sick man.

EPILOGUE: ANCIENT HISTORIES IN THE MODERN AGE

Modern men invented neither the Chinese medical fathers nor the idea of medical history in China. As my investigation of Needham's list of fathers reveals, the archive used by modern historians represents the legacy of ancient and medieval historiographical practices. Before the late first century BC, there is little evidence that anyone thought of the various techniques of healing as a single art form, one with a history of its own. Instead, what we find are isolated representations of exemplary healers, representations produced by a range of unrelated parties and toward different nonmedical ends. All this changed, due to the efforts of the imperial bibliographer, Liu Xiang. In compiling his list of exemplary healers, Liu Xiang provided later practitioners of the curative arts with the means to imagine themselves as part of a continuous past, stretching back to the dawn of time. Liu Xiang was not alone in shaping the modern historian's archive. As my discussion shows, later authors expanded upon Liu Xiang's list. They also reinterpreted the textual remnants of antiquity according to their own aims and preferences, thereby adding to the modern historian's stock of textual resources. The Chinese medical archive was thus the culmination of centuries of archival reordering and reconstruction.

My narrative is largely confined to the ancient and medieval period, but this does not mean that the story necessarily ended in the Song or Yuan dynasties. Undoubtedly, Ming and Qing scholars also contributed to the contour of the present archive. Indeed, future studies may investigate the ways in which the great imperial compilation projects and the evidential scholarship movement (*kaozheng* 考證) of late imperial China impinge upon current interpretations of the medical past.[1]

This epilogue does more than merely reflect upon the limitations of this study, however. Instead, I offer a final provocation, one that places the findings of the core chapters into a broader context. Toward this end, I return to the beginning of the book, and the twentieth-century retellings of the medical fathers. I attempt to situate these interpretations – or better yet, put them into perspective – within the long span of Chinese history. In this regard, my discussion runs counter to the current literature, which stresses that European ideologies, Marxism, scientism, and nationalism drove the modern historiography.[2] In contrast, I propose that while they betrayed European influence, the authors of this historiography had more in common with their ancient predecessors than generally supposed: they too stitched together pieces of existing stories in novel arrangements in order to imbue the medical fathers with fresh significance. In this way, my discussion challenges narratives of rupture by proposing that modern retellings of the Chinese past did *not* represent a break with earlier historiographical practice. On the contrary, such retellings represented the latest turn of the kaleidoscope – another iteration of a very long cycle of creation and destruction.

THE MODERN CONTEXT

It is imperative to place twentieth-century accounts in the context of the medical modernization that took place during the early twentieth century in China. In spite of the efforts of tireless European missionaries, who, by the mid-nineteenth century, had already been introducing Western medical practice and theory to Chinese converts for some time, Greater China was late to adopt such interventions.[3] And while some missionaries called attention to "China's appalling need for reform," a systematic or sustained effort to impose medical modernization came only after the first Sino-Japanese war (1894–5). Following an unexpected defeat by the Japanese, Chinese elites began to see the improvement of indigenous medicine as urgent. Reform-minded Chinese students began traveling in large numbers to Japan in order to study Western science, and particularly, Western medicine.[4]

In the first decades of the twentieth century, the tide turned decisively against the indigenous literate tradition, or what the elites of the time referred to as the old-style medicine. Such sentiments reflected the fact that the foreign-educated elite regarded the old-style medicine as "part of the corrupt and superstitious feudal culture holding back China's modernization."[5] In this regard, the remarks of one twentieth-century minister are revealing. He told a group of old-fashioned healers, "I have decided in the future to abolish Chinese medicine, and also not to use Chinese drugs."[6] One of the early founders of the Chinese Communist

Party expressed similar sentiments, lamenting, "Our doctors do not understand science. They not only know nothing of human anatomy, but also know nothing of the analysis of medicines; as for bacterial poisoning and infections, they have not even heard of them."[7] Most damning perhaps is the famous short story by the Japanese-educated Lu Xun 魯迅 (1881–1936), "Medicine" (*yao* 藥). In this, the old medicine served as a tangible symbol of the darkness and backwardness of traditional Chinese society. The story tells of a dying child, sick from consumption. In a futile, last-ditch effort to save the child, his parents prepare a traditional remedy: a bun dipped in the blood of an executed revolutionary.[8]

The years that spanned the decades between the fall of Qing and the establishment of the People's Republic of China witnessed the old medicine's decline in status. Such a decline was signaled by the sacking of palace physicians following the death of the Empress Dowager in 1908, a move that effectively ended centuries of imperial patronage for the learned tradition of medicine.[9] This was not the only, or even the most important, sign of change. That same year, a reform-minded provincial governor held the first medical licensing exam. The exam was notable for being the first recorded attempt to enforce licensing on all healers. The exam moreover required candidates to demonstrate knowledge of recent Western developments such as X-rays (which had only been discovered in 1895).[10] The founding of the Republican government after the 1911 revolution further contributed to the declining fortunes of Chinese medicine. As Bridie Andrews shows, the early Republican government was even more beholden to "scientism" than the late Qing state, for it created the Ministry of Health, which was dedicated to advancing the cause of Western medicine in China.[11]

In the first decades of the twentieth century, it seemed that the old-style medicine was slated for the dustbins of history, a casualty of the ascendancy of European science in China. In 1929, the National Board of Health even passed a resolution to abolish native practices of healing. As recounted by one prominent proponent, the committee's reasoning was as follows:

1. The old-style medicine of China adopts the doctrine of Yin and Yang principle, the five elements, the six atmospheres, the viscera and course of blood vessels. These are just *speculations* and have been proved to be inaccurate.
2. For diagnosis, the old-style physicians depend wholly on signs of the pulse. . . . *Such absurd theories are deceptive to themselves and their patients, and are as fallacious as astrology.*

3. Holding such views, the old-style practitioners cannot classify disease correctly or certify the causes of death, cannot combat epidemics, and cannot promote eugenics or racial betterment, and thus contribute to the people's welfare.
4. The *evolution of civilizations* is from the supernatural to the human, from the philosophical to the practical. While the government is educating the public as to the benefits of cleanliness and disinfection and a proper understanding of germs as the true cause of most diseases, the old-style practitioners preach wrong doctrines. . . . *These reactionary thoughts are the greatest hindrance to scientific progress.* [Emphases added.][12]

The influence of modern ideologies is clear in the author's assumptions about human societies: his supposition that history unfolded according to set stages, and his valuation of progress and scientific modernity. In addition, phrases such as eugenics and racial betterment speak to the sway that Social Darwinism held over the foreign-educated Chinese elite in the early twentieth century. Such language indicates the close connection between medical modernization and political strength in the minds of the cultural and ruling elite. For such elites, medical modernization was not only necessary for improving the health of Chinese society, but also crucial for Han racial survival.

Although ultimately unsuccessful, the proposed ban did have important ramifications for the old-styled medicine, as it prompted its thorough reevaluation – and some would say, its reinvention.[13] Some defenders of the tradition, now known as *Chinese* medicine, went to great lengths to make it appear more scientific. Responding to criticisms about the highly subjective quality of Chinese medical practice, some of the proponents strove for standardization and internal consistency in new textbooks.[14] Other men of similar persuasion, in contrast, evinced a sharp awareness of the low esteem that the metaphysical idiom of the classics enjoyed. So these supporters tiptoed gingerly around any reference to *yin*, *yang*, or the Five Phases.[15] Finally, some of the defenders adopted the epistemological framework of the opposition. Western-style doctors, including the leading proponent of the ban, Yu Yunxiu 余雲岫 (1879–1954), had denigrated Chinese medicine on the grounds that it was based on thousands of years of accumulated experience (*jingyan* 經驗) rather than scientific experiments. After 1929, however, practitioners of Chinese medicine co-opted the rhetoric of their opponents. In an attempt to salvage the reputation of Chinese medicine, such practitioners insisted that the real value of Chinese drugs lay not in a discredited metaphysical framework but rather upon the rich experiences of practitioners. Such a move reveals that while they had inverted their opponent's valuation of experience, the defenders had nevertheless accepted the epistemological platform created by proponents of Western science.[16]

The challenge posed by the ban also led to changes in healing practices. As Bridie Andrews points out, Chinese medicine today is largely synonymous with acupuncture. But in the early twentieth century acupuncture was a marginal practice, performed by members of the artisan class rather than by practitioners of the learned medicine. It took the efforts of a Japanese-trained physician, Cheng Dan'an 承淡安 (1899–1957), to bring this practice to prominence. Influenced by developments in Japan, Cheng redefined the acupuncture points described in ancient Chinese works, so as to align them with Western anatomical knowledge. At the same time, Cheng abandoned earlier practices that bore the stigma of superstition, including the practice of synchronizing the timing of acupuncture treatments with astrological calendars.[17] Cheng also abandoned the large metal needles and bodkins used to lance boils and to perform minor surgery in favor of the thin, filiform needles that are standard in acupuncture treatments today.[18]

The revival of acupuncture was not the only innovation that emerged in response to calls for medical modernization in China. The Communist era (1949–) also saw other important changes, including the mass publication of formerly secret family formulas and the push to require all practitioners to acquire training in Western medicine.[19] Indeed, the contemporary practice of Chinese medicine attests to such historical transformations. Acupuncturists today combine diverse understandings of the body and technologies to treat biomedical conditions such as Parkinson's disease and menopause.[20] And Chinese-styled healers connect their clinical encounters with works attributed to Huangfu Mi's fathers of medicine.[21] Such changes disclose the extent to which European science and ideology reconfigured Chinese medical practice in the twentieth century.

THE NEW HISTORIES

The challenge posed by Western science not only influenced the practice and status of Chinese medicine; it also stimulated the writing of new histories of healing. Before we take a look at the contents and designs of these histories, it would be worthwhile to say a few words about the backgrounds of the leading twentieth-century historians. As shall be demonstrated, the first generations of historians were a motley bunch, divided in education and experience, as well as motive. Such differences notwithstanding, their accounts of the medical past reflected the influence of both European ideologies and premodern Chinese traditions of historiography.

THE HISTORIANS AND THEIR MOTIVES

Some of the authors of these new histories were participants of the National Medicine Movement. These included Xie Guan 謝觀 (1880–1950), who published in 1935 the *Origins and Development of Chinese Medicine* (*Zhongguo yixue yuanliu lun* 中國醫學源流論). Xie had ties to a prestigious medical lineage in Southeast China that produced famous healers and respected authors for centuries.[22] Xie was also an important defender and reformer of Chinese medicine. He helped to establish a Chinese medical college and administered licensing exams for medical practitioners. Despite such efforts to update medical practice, Xie remained a conservative figure. As Andrews points out, Xie avoided using Western medical terminology, lest he become a "slave" to Western culture.[23] As with Xie Guan, Chen Cunren 陳存仁 (1908–90) was a Chinese-style healer and a leading figure in the Chinese medicine movement. According to Andrews, Chen played a major role in coordinating the congress and delegations that successfully thwarted the proposed ban.[24] Decades later, Chen would publish his own history of Chinese medicine (*Zhongguo yixueshi* 中國醫學史; 1968), a work characterized by its copious use of illustrations of ancient healers.[25]

In contrast, other authors remained within the orbit of the medical modernizers. This includes Chen Bangxian, widely regarded as the father of modern Chinese medical history and an early leader in the Institute of Chinese Medicine in Beijing. Chen had been the disciple of Ding Fubao 丁福寶 (1875–1952), an advocate for the scientization of Chinese medicine.[26] Another of the early historians was Fan Xingzhun (1906–98), who also held a leadership role in the early Institute of Medicine. Like Ding, Fan sympathized with the cause of medical modernization[27] and took a critical attitude toward members of the National Medicine Movement. As Sean Lei shows, Fan rejected the claim that Chinese medicine should be preserved because it reflected China's national essence. The view of Chinese medicine as a uniquely Chinese phenomenon, Fan argued, revealed ignorance of its heterogeneous roots. As he took pains to demonstrate, Chinese medicine had incorporated elements of foreign cultures for centuries before the coming of European science and technology in the nineteenth century.[28]

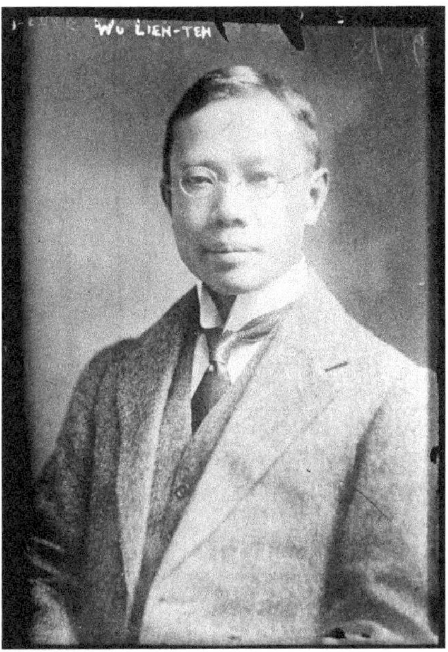

Figure 17 Wu Lien-teh, a medical modernizer, proponent of the 1929 ban on Chinese medicine, and coauthor of the *History of Chinese Medicine: Being a Chronicle of Medical Happenings in China from Ancient Times to the Present Period* (1932).

Source: Reproduced from Bain News Service (ca. 1910 and ca. 1915).

Some of the first modern historians trained abroad were outspoken opponents of Chinese medicine, who campaigned for its abolition. Take the case of Wu Lien-teh 伍連德 (1879–1960), the Cambridge-educated physician from colonial Malaya, who spent his formative years in England (see Figure 17). By his own admission, Wu's command of the Chinese language was rudimentary and his knowledge of Chinese history shaky, or as he put it, "Although of Chinese parentage, I could barely write my name in Chinese characters, let alone read a newspaper in the Chinese language."[29] In the first decades of the twentieth century, Wu worked for the late Qing court (sending his communications in English). Thanks to his efforts to control outbreaks of pneumonic plague in Manchuria from 1910 to 1911, Wu became a celebrated and influential figure in China. Around this time, he also found himself at loggerheads with the old-style healers, and so became a leading figure in the proposal to abolish native medicine. In a memoir published a year before his death in 1960, Wu complained that the old-fashioned medicine not only survived but continued to thrive – in spite of his best efforts to abolish and restrict its practice. "In spite of government laws and restrictions," he wrote, "the native herbalists continue to function and contribute to the high incidence of mortality for childbirth, infantile diseases and infections."[30] Such misgivings notwithstanding, Wu wrote the *History of Chinese Medicine: Being a Chronicle of Medical Happenings in China from Ancient Times to the Present Period* (1932). Almost a thousand pages long, this tome set forth the first English-language treatment of Chinese medical history. It had been inspired by Wu's discovery that Western historians of medicine had overlooked China. Sensing that China deserved a place within the world history of medicine, Wu then wrote his history with Wang Jimin 王吉民 (also known as Wong K. Chimin; 1889–1972), a Western-style doctor from Hong Kong and the author of *Medical Innovations in Historical China* (*Zhongguo lidai yixue zhi faming* 中國歷代醫學之發明).[31]

SIGNS OF EUROPEAN INFLUENCE

The influence of modernity is evident in the new image of the medical fathers. In this respect, Hua Tuo (d. ca. AD 208), a legendary healer, provides a prime example. As I have only mentioned Hua Tuo in passing, a few words about premodern treatments of this ubiquitous figure are in order. The earliest surviving description of him appeared in a historical chronicle, the *Record of the Three Kingdoms* (*Sanguo zhi* 三國志; comp. ca. AD 290). This third-century chronicler treated his readers to the choicest cuts of legend so as to create a memorable image of the figure. These included fantastic tales about Hua Tuo's skills at healing: sick patients cured by garlic purees that induced the vomiting of snakes; women who gave birth to stone fetuses months after live deliveries; and, last but not least, a mysterious anesthesia used by the famed healer to render patients unconscious before surgery.[32] The chronicler, however, did not stop with his descriptions of Hua Tuo's curative prowess; he also rehearsed stories that portrayed Hua Tuo as a transcendent (*xian* 仙), or extraordinarily long-lived – if not deathless – being.[33] Toward this end, the chronicler stressed Hua Tuo's knowledge of calisthenics and alchemy,[34] knowledge that the healer purportedly had transmitted to his disciples.[35]

Interestingly, Hua Tuo's image did not change much over the long course of China's imperial period. Later accounts closely followed his third-century portrait, stressing both his surgical prowess and skills at extending life.[36] In fact, authors of medieval and late imperial compendia gave as much weight to Hua Tuo's knowledge of the arts of transcendence as to his surgical prowess. One twelfth-century author summarized Hua Tuo's achievements in the following way: "He possessed a penetrating knowledge of medical formulas, and he was apt at the arts of nourishing life, so when he was over a hundred years old, he had the countenance of someone in his prime." The people of his age, the author added, "regarded Hua Tuo as a transcendent."[37]

In the twentieth century, however, Hua Tuo's image underwent a makeover, as modern historians made much of his purported surgical skills. In *Medical Innovations*, Wang argued that the records of Hua Tuo's surgeries proved that the Chinese had discovered and perfected the use of anesthesia – long before its discovery in Europe in the mid-nineteenth century.[38] Hua Tuo's surgery also proved to be a subject of great interest to other twentieth-century historians. Wu and Wang devoted space in their English-language history to speculating about the potential ingredients in Hua Tuo's mysterious preparation. There, they guessed that the "effervescing powder of Hua Tuo," along with the "narcotic wine of Bian Que" employed "datura alba, rhododendron sinesa, jasmine sambac, and various aconites."[39]

Twentieth-century historians did more than emphasize Hua Tuo's surgical prowess, however. To give this medieval figure a thoroughly scientific makeover, they also downplayed his associations with the arts of transcendence, considered by many to be superstition. Chen Cunren's *History of Chinese Medicine* passed over in silence Hua Tuo's pursuit of transcendence and focused exclusively on his curative skills. Although he disclosed Hua Tuo's "discovery" of calisthenics, Chen interpreted the discovery as a sign that the ancient healer regarded exercise as the foundation of good health. In this way, Chen distanced Hua Tuo from the pursuit of superlongevity or immortality.[40] Most telling, perhaps, was Li Jingwei's treatment of this healer. An important historian, Li claimed that Hua Tuo's emphasis on calisthenics revealed that the ancient healer promoted "preventive" health care. More improbably, Li insisted that Hua Tuo was different from the quacks of his age, who had promoted the use of mineral elixirs. This last characterization of Hua Tuo, it goes without saying, required some cherry picking on Li's part.[41] At the very least, it necessitated a selective reading of the textual record, one that overlooked the fact that prominent medieval authors, including a celebrated authority on pharmacopeia, had credited Hua Tuo and his disciples with discovering various elixirs of immortality.[42]

Hua Tuo was not the only exemplary healer from antiquity who underwent a facelift. More radical, I think, was the remaking of Attendant

He (Chapter 1). As we saw earlier, premodern authors had extolled this healer for his deft understanding of the numinous realm. Yet this reputation hardly deterred the father of modern Chinese historiography; Chen Bangxian characterized Attendant He as the spokesman of a naturalist philosophy. According to Chen, Attendant He's prognosis of Lord Jin signaled medicine's rejection of religious conceptions of illness and a "split with superstitious healers."[43] Similarly, in the *Short History of Chinese Medicine*, Fan Xingzhun highlighted the fact that the healer framed illness solely in terms of *qi*, a move that Fan read as a sign that medicine "had already broken through the barriers of religion and superstition."[44]

Zhang Ji (see Chapter 5) also acquired a new persona in modern histories. In their collaborative *History of Medicine in China*, Wu and Wang went so far as to proclaim Zhang Ji the "Hippocrates of China."[45] They noted that the *Cold Damage Disorders* omitted all references to the pernicious *yin yang* or Five Phases metaphysics, often blamed by modernizers for having inhibited the development of science in China. The work, they added, was eminently practical, being grounded solely in Zhang Ji's own experience and firsthand observations. In this connection, the authors noted, "Diseases were studied more from a clinical standpoint, emphasis being laid on the physical signs, symptoms, and causes of an illness, the methods of treatment and the action of drugs, rather than on the theories of disease as in former times."[46]

SIMILARITIES TO ANCIENT AND MEDIEVAL HISTORIES

Although they betrayed the influence of European ideologies and modern science, twentieth-century retellings also exhibited striking continuities with the earlier historiography. Consider Chen Cunren's *History of Chinese Medicine*. In many regards, this work was not different from earlier accounts that adorned the prefaces and postfaces of most imperial treatises, for Chen opened by reciting the accomplishments of bygone healers: the Divine Husbandman ("The Earliest Chinese Herbalist"), the Yellow Emperor ("The Pioneer of Chinese Medical Science"), Bian Que ("The First Acupuncturist and Doctor"), Hua Tuo ("The First Surgeon of the World"), and Zhang Ji ("The Foremost Chinese Physician of the Second Century"), among others.[47] Many of the stories Chen Cunren cited were identical to those of earlier histories. Like Huangfu Mi (see Chapter 4), Chen Cunren credited the Divine Husbandman with tasting (or "testing") all of the plants to identify their curative properties, and celebrated the Yellow Emperor for discovering with his ministers the secrets of the human body.[48] Chen furthermore attributed Zhang Ji's decision to write his treatise to the devastating epidemic that wiped out the ancient healer's family.[49]

Other modern histories also reveal signs of influence from the ancient historiography. Most remarkable is the case of Wu and Wang's English-language history of medicine (I say remarkable because of Wu's illiteracy in Chinese). There, the influence of an older, classical historiography is nevertheless clear from their treatment of ancient medicine, a sign perhaps of Wang's influence over his more famous collaborator. In their preface, Wu and Wang commemorated the exemplary figures of antiquity. "The Han dynasty, which is considered the most glorious epoch in Chinese medical history," they wrote, "was rendered especially memorable from the fact that during this period there lived the Granary Master, Zhang Ji, and Hua Tuo."[50] Not satisfied with merely commemorating a handful of figures, Wu and Wang also recited the history of medicine from the beginning of time. In a chapter entitled, "Founders of Chinese Medicine," they enumerated the purported deeds of archaic figures, who they treated as mythical beings. In subsequent chapters – "Famous Ancient Physicians" and "The Great Trio" – they remembered the figures who lived during the various stages of more recent antiquity: Yi Yin, Attendant He, Bian Que, Chunyu Yi, Hua Tuo, and Zhang Ji. And like countless medical authors before them, Wu and Wang treated all of these figures as historical personages.

Besides the focus on exemplary figures, twentieth-century historians shared with premodern scholars common strategies for giving old figures new significance. For evidence of the enduring quality of what Mario Biagioli calls the logic of the graft,[51] let us see how modern historians arrived at their interpretations of the medical fathers. Take Attendant He, whose current image as a naturalist is opposite of his earlier reputation as an expert of the numinous realm. As we saw in Chapter 1, the figure in the *Tradition of Zuo* had enjoyed more than one reincarnation before the twentieth century. In preimperial texts, chroniclers treated him as a rhetorical device, a doppelgänger added to stories for purposes of narrative intensification. Yet as we saw in Chapter 4, Liu Xiang had reinvented the ancient figure as an actual personage during the Han dynasty by extracting him from a political parable and inserting him into a story about the progress of the curative arts over time. In this way, Liu Xiang paved the way for the episode – or better still, some parts of it – to be read as a literal medical happening. When he painted Attendant He as the vanguard of a new naturalistic medicine, Chen Bangxian similarly had only to cut out the same passages from the ancient sources used by Liu Xiang. And for the most part, Chen's story about Attendant He was virtually indistinguishable from earlier accounts – with one difference. In recapping the story about Attendant He's visit to the state of Jin, Chen omitted the prophecy about the minister's imminent death, an omission necessary for Chen's story about a historic victory of rationalism over superstition.[52] Though novel, Chen's interpretation of Attendant He was hardly created from nothing, being predicated on Liu Xiang's previous reinvention of the figure as a historical personage.

The reevaluation of Zhang Ji proceeded by similar routes. Zhang Ji's reputation as a forward-thinking physician also resulted from modern historians repurposing existing textual matter. To outfit Zhang Ji with a new persona, such historians took pieces of the preface to the *Cold Damage Disorders* and inserted them into a new story: one about the role played by careful, firsthand observations in what they now sold as a clinical encounter.[53] This penchant for creating mash-ups of Zhang Ji, however, was hardly unprecedented. As seen in Chapter 5, Zhang Ji's tragic persona was a *bricolage*, an artifact of centuries of editors rearranging and recycling pieces of textual fragments. The remaking of Zhang Ji along ideological lines – evident in the presentation of the figure as a *scientific* healer – had been anticipated by Song and Yuan literati. Such literati had previously replaced a still earlier image of the figure as a wonderworker so as to align him with their ideals and aspirations.

HISTORIES PAST AND FUTURE

So how does one account for the resonances between modern and ancient histories? As discussed previously, the modern historiography in English and Chinese bears testimony to the imprint of Western ideologies. Such ideologies, which included scientism and Marxism, evidently shaped the modern meanings attributed to the medical fathers. At the same time, such histories also attest to the persistent influence of indigenous conceptual categories and historiographical practices.[54] Like Huangfu Mi and other medieval scholars, twentieth-century historians intoned the names of the medical fathers, elaborating upon their deeds and remembering their contributions. And by weaving bits and pieces of myth into their stories about the past, historians such as Chen Bangxian and Wu Lien-teh imparted the fathers with a new range of meanings.

In part, one may explain the resonances between modern and ancient accounts by the collaborations that occurred between historians trained

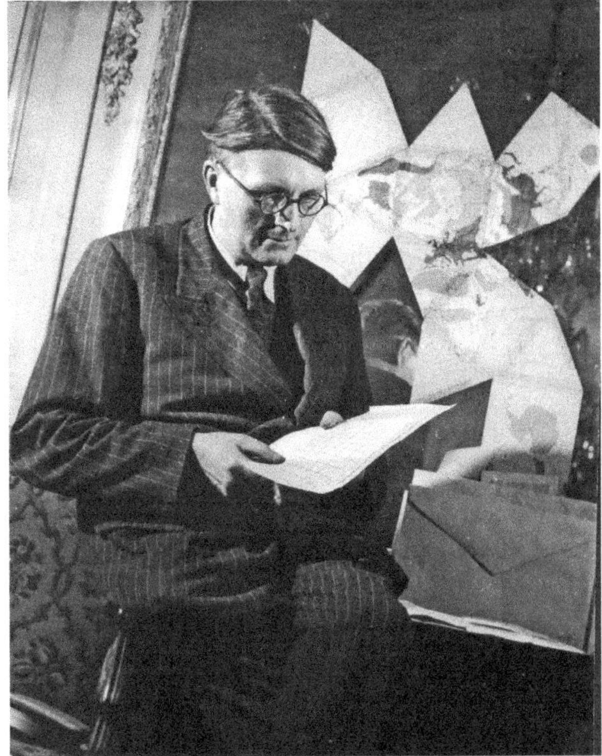

Figure 18 Joseph Needham, a pioneer in the history of Chinese medicine.
Source: Courtesy of the Needham Research Institute.

in the West and those versed in the indigenous tradition of scholarship – the collaborations that have been highlighted by Thomas Trautmann and other scholars writing against the postcolonial vein.[55] In the Chinese case, collaboration occurred not between colonial Orientalists and native Indian pandits, but rather between European-educated historians and physicians, on the one hand, and scholars trained in the Chinese classics, on the other. For evidence of such a phenomenon, one need not look beyond the first generation of European-educated historians and physicians. As noted previously, the Cambridge-educated Wu Lien-teh wrote the first English-language history of Chinese medicine with Wang Jimin, who had the benefit of classical training. Similarly, Joseph Needham wrote *Science and Civilization* with Chinese-educated coauthors, most famously Lu Gwei-djen (see Figure 18).[56] In the preface to *Celestial Lancets*, Needham and Lu moreover acknowledged their conversations with a broad array of Chinese colleagues, including Chen Bangxian and Wang Jimin.[57]

One may also account for the resonances between ancient and modern histories by the fact that twentieth-century scholars used the same materials as their forebears. To be sure, it is tempting to treat such materials as mere "content," or the raw matter with which to flesh out a European theoretical skeleton. Yet I would hasten to note that these materials – be they parcels of ancient texts or lists of exemplary healers – were anything but raw data. By the time they reached the desks of twentieth-century historians, such materials had undergone centuries, even millennia, of processing. The materials thus arrived laden with the assumptions of earlier generations of anthologists, editors, and medical historians. Such assumptions determined *which* figures populated Chinese medical history – in other words, who represented the proper subject of historical inquiry. These assumptions also governed what counted as medical history: *which* editions were considered definitive or reliable, and *which* happenings represented critical moments in the formation of the medical tradition.

When he sat down to compose his history of medicine, Chen Bangxian found that much of the interpretative and archival spadework had already been done for him. Take his *Record of Chinese Medical Personalities* (*Zhongguo yixue renming zhi* 中國醫學人名誌; 1956), an encyclopedic collection of the biographies of all known healers before the twentieth century.[58] For this task, Chen and his collaborator appropriated the materials supplied by earlier anthologies from the medieval or late imperial period. When describing Zhang Ji's career, for example, they drew upon the capsule biography of the famed healer preserved in a Ming gazetteer, a source also used by the Qing editors of an important medical compilation.[59] When writing the entry on Huangfu Mi (see Chapter 6), Chen and his collaborator similarly excerpted the description of the third-century man found in a sixteenth-century source.[60] Chen's source, it turns out, had been previously lifted from an earlier anthology that emphasized Huangfu Mi's editorial contributions over his knowledge of mineral poisoning. For this reason, Chen's anthology promoted the pedantic image of Huangfu Mi over the earlier one of him as a chronic sick man. As such, it reproduced the rhetorical maneuvers and agendas of scholars living in the eleventh century.

The materials marshaled by modern and ancient historians thus represented a zone of contact for European-educated scholars, who mixed their ideologies with ancient Chinese historiographical practice. When

Joseph Needham took up the writing of Chinese medical history beginning in 1954, he not only had the assistance of Chinese collaborators, but also the accumulated efforts of thousands of years of scholarship. This much can be gleaned from his bibliography, which discloses that he and Lu availed themselves to a wide range of resources transmitted through the ages, including medieval anthologies like the *Discourses on Medicine* and the *Primer of Famous Healers through the Ages*.[61] Viewed from this perspective, Needham's interpretation of the archive was both enabled and constrained by earlier reorderings. Or to borrow Marx's turn of phrase, Needham may very well have made his own history of Chinese medicine, but he did not make it as he pleased.

An investigation into the medical fathers takes us far from an indictment of modernity. Certainly, scholars have rightfully criticized twentieth-century retellings of Chinese medical history for their modern biases. Yet this perspective, I would argue, does not reveal everything. By tracing the changing faces of the medical fathers over time, this book proffers an alternative narrative, one that illuminates the influence of earlier generations of editors, healers, and medical authors. In so doing, the *Art of Medicine* demonstrates that the efforts of previous generations inform the contents of modern histories, including this one. Like the classical scholars, medical modernizers, and Marxists who have come before me, I have told my story through the medical fathers. Toward this end, I revisited the episodes found in disparate genres and collections, scrutinizing the definitive versions left behind by Song scholars for signs of tampering and creative editing. Like Huangfu Mi and Needham, I too am a *bricoleur*. Having appropriated the materials made for other purposes, I used them to narrate a history that reflects the concerns of my time and place. And for this reason, the *Art of Medicine* bears testimony to the resilience of ancient ways of knowing. It shows that the historiographical practices of antiquity are not gone; such practices live on, embedded in the very fabric of our modern retellings.

APPENDIX: A PROBLEMATIC PREFACE

Most scholars have assumed that the preface to the *Cold Damage Disorders* was written by the historical Zhang Ji. This appendix, which provides the supporting documentation for the technical arguments of Chapter 5, challenges the received view. I argue that the contents of the preface evolved over time. Toward this end, I examine the contents of the current preface to the *Cold Damage Disorders* (hereafter the current preface) and related materials in sources dating to the Sui or Tang dynasties, the early Song, and the eleventh century. All of the sources encompassed by my discussion have been set forth in Table 6. In addition, I include a full transcription and translation of the current version of the preface at the end of this appendix.

I am not the first person to question the provenance of the preface. Others, including Wang Pinxian 王聘賢 and his coauthors, argued in 1982 that the text was spurious.[1] While the views of Wang and colleagues have not been influential, other scholars have voiced their suspicions about the preface. More recently, Qian Chaochen 錢超塵 argues that the later portions of the text contain interpolations of extraneous materials taken from Sun Simiao's corpus and commentarial matter. Qian's assessment is based on his comparison of the current preface with the Kangping 康平 edition, which will be discussed in the following text.[2] Still others, Chen Senhe 陳森和 and Ouyang Yu'e 歐陽玉娥, have voiced additional concerns. Chen and Ouyang convincingly show the existence of interpolations into the preface by revealing the close resemblance between the preface by Sun Simiao, on the one hand, and the current preface attributed to Zhang, on the other. Like the current preface, Sun's preface discusses his motivations for studying medicine: his desire to help his relatives and neighbors who were suffering from the affliction of illness. His remark – "I grieve for those who have died prematurely"

Table 6 *Sources for the Appendix*

Name	Date	Site	Format	Contents
Cold Damage Disorders	Sui Dynasty	Dunhuang	Manuscript	Parallels to the *Cold Damage Disorders*, in three manuscript fragments
Sun Zhenren's Formulas Worth a Thousand Gold (hereafter *Sun Zhenren's Formulas*)	Tang Dynasty	Japan	Manuscript	Two parallels to the current preface, one listed as the words of Zhang Ji and a work called the *Treatise on Formulas* 方論
Cold Damage Disorders of the Kangzhi Era 康治本傷寒論 (hereafter Kangzhi edition)	Ca. 805	Japan	Manuscript	Partial copy of the *Cold Damage Disorders* without a preface
Imperial Review of the Era of Great Peace 太平御覽 (hereafter *Imperial Review*)	977–83	n/a	Print edition	Quotations from a preface to the *Formulas of Zhang Zhongjing* 張仲景方論序
Gao Jichong 高繼沖本 edition of the *Cold Damage Disorders*	992	n/a	Printed	Partial copy of the *Cold Damage Disorders* without preface
Cold Damage Disorders of the Kangping Era 康平本傷寒論 (hereafter Kangping edition)	1060	Japan	Manuscript	Partial copy of the *Cold Damage Disorders* with a preface
Cold Damage Disorders found in the *Additional Formulas Worth a Thousand Gold* 千金翼方 (hereafter the Sun Simiao version)	Eleventh century	n/a	Print edition of Tang dynasty work	Partial copy of the *Cold Damage Disorders* without a preface
Preface to the Cold Damage Disorders (hereafter current preface)	1065	n/a	Print edition	Preface in full
Discourses on Medicine	Twelfth through thirteenth century	n/a	Print edition	Quotations from a preface to the *Formulas of Zhang Zhongjing*

(*tong yaowang zhi you e* 痛夭枉之幽厄)[3] – resonates with the statement in the current preface to the *Cold Damage Disorders:* "pained by those who could not be rescued from their untimely deaths" (*shang hengyao zhi moqiu* 傷横夭之莫救). This is not the only similarity. Chen and Ouyang also find the passage that immediately follows the discussion of the epidemic to be similar to a passage in Sun Simiao:

Sun Simiao	Kangping edition preface
乃博採羣經。刪裁繁重。務在簡易。以為備急千金要 方一部。凡三十卷。雖不能究盡病源。但使留意於斯者。亦思過半矣。	博采衆方。為傷寒卒病論。 雖未能盡愈諸病。庶可以見病知源。若能尋余所集。思過半矣。
I have selected broadly from the multitude of classics, cutting what was wordy and superfluous. My task resided in simplifying [existing material], so as to make a text, the *Formulas Worth a Thousand Gold*, altogether in thirty rolls. Although the resultant work does not exhaust the causes of all illness, one has only to pay attention to it to know more than most.[4]	I have selected widely from the multitudes of formulas. All these have been used to make the *Treatise on Cold Damage Disorders and the Miscellaneous Illnesses*. Although the resultant work cannot cure all illnesses, it can probably be used to apprehend the illness and understand its cause. If one is able to use what I have collected, then they will know more than most.[5]

The possibility that lines from Sun Simiao's corpus may have been intermingled into the text of the *Cold Damage Disorders* is hardly surprising. Portions of the *Cold Damage Disorders*, in fact, circulated as part of Sun Simiao's corpus.[6]

There is an additional reason to question the current preface's provenance. The contents and ordering of the preface changed repeatedly over the centuries. To see this, let us review the different manuscript editions of the text.

SUI AND TANG MANUSCRIPTS

At first glance, Tang dynasty manuscripts would seem to confirm that Zhang Ji was the author of the current preface. This is because of nine parallels found in *Sun Zhenren's Formulas Worth a Thousand Gold* (*Sun Zhenren qianjin fang* 孫真人千金方). For ease of discussion, I will refer to the nine parallels as A–I. These labels do not reflect the order in which they appear in the current preface. Instead, they mark the temporal strata of the passages. Passages that appear in earlier sources will be referred to

Table 7 *Components of the Preface to the Cold Damage Disorders*

Passage	Sources	Contents
A	*Sun Zhenren's Formulas*; current preface; Kangping ms.	First polemic about Zhang Ji's contemporaries who have neglected the arts of healing and their misplaced priorities
B	*Sun Zhenren's Formulas*; current preface; Kangping ms.	Complaints about contemporaries who do not succeed in public life and who neglect the health of the body
C	*Sun Zhenren's Formulas*; current preface; Kangping ms.	Observation that such contemporaries are rendered helpless when ill
D	*Sun Zhenren's Formulas*; current preface; Kangping ms.	Observation that such contemporaries are endangered by their illnesses
E	*Sun Zhenren's Formulas*; current preface; Kangping ms.	Observation that such contemporaries succumb to specious methods or quack healers when sick
F	*Sun Zhenren's Formulas;* current preface; Kangping ms.	The working of the Five Phases
G	*Sun Zhenren's Formulas*	Importance of the ideal perceptual agent for perceiving subtle phenomena
G_1	Current preface and Kangping ms.	Importance of the ideal perceptual agent for perceiving subtle phenomena (quotation from *Book of Changes*)
H	*Sun Zhenren's Formulas*; current preface; Kangping ms.	An additional polemic about contemporary healers and their specious techniques
I	*Sun Zhenren's Formulas*; current preface; Kangping ms.	Limited perspective and abilities of contemporary healers
J	*Imperial Review*	Story about Zhang Ji's disciple
K	Current preface; Kangping ms.	Two stories about Bian Que
L	Current preface; Kangping ms.	Adversities faced by contemporaries
M	Current preface; Kangping ms.	Additional polemic about contemporaries with frivolous pursuits
N	Current preface; Kangping ms.	Dangers faced by contemporaries
O	Current preface; Kangping ms.	Epidemic story
P	Current preface; Kangping ms.	Description of the *Cold Damage Disorders*
Q	Current preface; Kangping ms.	History of medicine from antiquity to Han dynasty
R	Current preface; Kangping ms.	Final remarks
S	Current preface	Description of sources for *Cold Damage Disorders*

with letters from the beginning of the alphabet. All of the passages discussed are shown in Table 7.

Taken together, the nine parallels make up nearly one-half of the contents of the current preface. Interestingly, the story about the epidemic, which is prominently highlighted in the current preface, is absent from any of these.

A closer look at the nine parallels as they appear in *Sun Zhenren's Formulas*, however, suggests the need for caution. To begin with, none of the nine are cited as coming from any preface whatsoever. *Sun Zhenren's Formulas* quotes A, B, C, D, and E as the words of Zhang Ji. In contrast, F, G, H, and I are quoted as being from a work called the *Treatise on Formulas* (*Fanglun* 方論). Viewed from this perspective, it is unclear whether the nine parallels were originally part of the same text, let alone a preface by Zhang Ji.[7]

Making matters worse, the other Sui and Tang manuscripts containing parallels to the *Cold Damage Disorders* provide no trace of a preface. This includes the sizable manuscript discovered in Japan (the Kangzhi 康治 manuscript), dating to the early ninth century, as well as the three fragments recovered from the Dunhuang caves, and a version of the manuscript found in the *Supplemental Formulas*, attributed to Sun Simiao of the Tang dynasty.[8]

EARLY SONG (TENTH CENTURY)

The first time that anyone mentions a preface attributed to Zhang Ji is during the late tenth century. The *Imperial Review of the Era of Great Peace* (hereafter *Imperial Review*; comp. 977–83), in fact, quotes a passage from a work referred to as the *Preface to the Formulas of Zhang Zhongjing* (*Zhang Zhongjing fanglun xu* 張仲景方論序). The *Formulas of Zhang Zhongjing* is believed by many scholars to have represented the larger corpus from which the current version of the *Cold Damage Disorders* derived.[9] I will refer to this quotation from the preface as J.[10]

Although it confirms the existence of a preface, J does not support the assumption that the current preface was written by the historical Zhang Ji. First of all, there is no overlap between J and the current preface, and J is quite different in terms of content and style. To see this, we must look more closely at J, which discusses Zhang Ji's disciple, Wei Fan 衛汎: "Wei Fan was fond of the arts of the healer, and in his youth, he became the pupil of Zhang Ji. . . ."[11] The text then proceeds to list all of the works by Wei Fan. What is worth drawing from this is the way that Zhang Ji is referred to in the third person in J, in contrast to the current preface, which is written in the first person. In terms of content, J is also a mismatch with the current preface, as the latter makes no mention of the author's broader social circle. Due to such discrepancies, it seems unlikely that J was ever part of the same text as the current preface.

In addition, the preface is missing from the Gao Jichong 高繼沖 version of the *Cold Damage Disorders*, which was printed for the first time in 992 as part of the imperial compendium, the *Formulas for Sagehood and Compassion in the Era of Great Peace* (*Taiping Shenghui fang* 太平聖惠方).[12]

EDITION OF 1060

Another Japanese edition (the Kangping) was discovered by scholars in 1937. The text is dated to 1060 based on internal evidence, with additional notations dating to 1346.[13] Some controversy exists as to the dates of the contents of this edition. Based on what might look at first glance to be a pattern of taboo avoidance and assumptions about when Chinese manuscripts arrived in Japan, Qian Chaochen puts the date of the manuscript between the Sui dynasty and 805. Qian's arguments, however, falter upon careful examination.[14] The same pattern of taboo avoidance is found in a version of the *Cold Damage Disorders* based on Song printed manuscripts. What is more, most historians believe that Chinese manuscripts arrived in Japan continuously until the end of the Yuan period. In contrast, Chen and Ouyang have recently proposed a late-Tang date for the Kangping version. They have convincingly shown that portions of Sun Simiao's corpus have been inserted into the preface to the Kangping edition.[15]

The differences from the earlier two versions may be summarized in the following ways: The contents in the tenth-century version – in particular J, which once contained descriptions of Zhang Ji's disciple – have been removed. I say removed rather than lost because we find quotations of J and other parts of the preface to the *Formulas of Zhang Zhongjing* in an anthology dating between the twelfth or thirteenth century.[16]

This is not the only difference. The sequence that the parallels follow in *Sun Zhenren's Formulas* is different from the Kangping edition, as shown in Figure 19.

More importantly, we find the addition of new content. The story about the epidemic, for example, has been added. We also find that F, H, and I – found in Sun Simiao but not listed as the words of Zhang

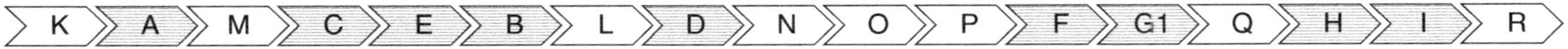

K A M C E B L D N O P F G1 Q H I R

Figure 19 The sequence of the Kangping edition, ca. AD 1060. The cells in shade represent materials found in the Tang edition of Sun Simiao. Everything else is found in later manuscripts.

Source: Figure drawn by author.

K A C E B L D M N O S P F G1 Q H I R

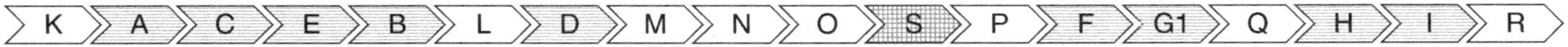

Figure 20 The current preface of the *Cold Damage Disorders*, ca. AD 1065. The cell marked S represents material that was not part of the main text in the Kangping edition of 1060.

Source: Figure drawn by author.

Ji – have been included in the same document. G has also been substituted with a similar passage, which I will call G_1. F, G_1, H, and I have, moreover, been set off from the rest of the text. Some modern scholars interpret this as a sign that F, G_1, H, and I are to be read as commentary. While plausible, this is not the only possible explanation. One could also argue that F, G_1, H, and I were regarded by the copier merely as another text. This is because the copier was careful to differentiate between the commentary and classic, as he would use *zhu* 注 (commentary) and *jing* 經 (classic) to mark off the boundaries of the text. In this case, we do not find F, G_1, H, and I marked off as commentary with *zhu*.

EDITION OF 1065

It is only in the mid-eleventh century that we see the current preface in its contemporary form.[17] For the most part, the current preface is similar to the Kangping edition, although there are several differences worth noting. First, the smaller differences: whereas the Kangping edition omits the description of the *Cold Damage Disorders*, the current version includes a statement about the text being in sixteen rolls. Second, the sequence of the preface is different, as indicated by Figure 20. We also see the firm integration of A, B, C, D, and E, on the one hand, with F, G_1, H, and I, on the other. Finally and most strikingly, we see the inclusion of S. The move to include S, which describes the author's sources for the *Cold Damage Disorders*, is worth expanding upon. Although S is only formally incorporated into the main text of the 1065 edition, S appears in the Kangping edition – where it is formally marked as commentary. The move to include S suggests that the Song editors had mistaken commentary for the main text, an observation that squares with the present evidence.

Taken together, the facts indicate that the current preface evolved substantially over the centuries. As we have already seen, the contents of the preface associated with Zhang Ji appear to have changed over time, with passages having been added, removed, and rearranged. Equally troubling is clear evidence that commentarial matter had been intermingled into the main text in the process of transmission. Finally, we find signs that portions of Sun Simiao's corpus managed to creep into the main text. All these factors undermine our confidence in the current version of the preface – the story about the epidemic in particular – as original to the third century.

TRANSLATION OF THE CURRENT PREFACE

	Passage	Translation
K	論曰：余每覽越人入虢之診。望齊侯之色，未嘗不慨然歎其才秀也。	The *Treatise* says: "I am always moved to sigh with admiration each time I recall how Bian Que entered the state of Guo and examined [the crown prince] or how he [determined the fact of illness] merely by gazing from afar at the appearance of the Lord of Qi."
A	怪當今居世之士。曾不留神醫藥。精究方術，上以療君親之疾，下以救貧賤之厄，中以保長身全，以養其性，但競逐榮勢，企踵權豪，孜孜汲汲，惟名利是務，崇飾其末，忽棄其本，華其外，而悴其內．皮之不存。毛將安附焉。	I thus consider strange the gentlemen of my age, who are not mindful of the art of medicine. They do not concentrate on the study of the arts to treat the illnesses of their lords and parents above, nor to deliver from disaster the poor and humble below, nor do they even seek in the middle to preserve the body and complete their life spans, or to nourish life. On the contrary, such men compete for glory, standing on tiptoes around the powerful and influential, busying themselves in their midst. And if it benefits their reputations, such men will serve; consequently, they adorn the ends, disregarding and forsaking the root; embellishing that without while allowing that within to wither. But if the skin no longer exists, how can the hair be attached to it?
C	卒然遭邪風之氣，嬰非常之疾，患及禍至，而方震慄，	When they are suddenly stricken with the *qi* of a wind pathology or encounter some strange illness, they tremble with fear as the calamity befalls them.
E	降志屈節，欽望巫祝，告窮歸天，束手受敗，賫百年之壽命，持至貴之重器，委付凡醫，恣其所措，咄嗟嗚呼！厥身已斃，神明消滅，變為異物，幽潛重泉，徒為啼泣，痛夫！舉世昏迷，莫能覺悟，不惜其命，若是輕生，彼何榮勢之云哉！	At a loss with respect to their aims, they bend their principles, paying their respects to witches and invocators, making announcements and entrusting themselves to Heaven. With their hands bound, they accept the calamity that has befallen them. In other cases, they regard a life span of a century as a precious commodity. They thus consign themselves to the care of quack healers, doing as they are instructed. Is this not lamentable! When the body has been killed, the illumination of the spirit extinguished, and the body transformed into a corpse, such men will be submerged in the darkness of the netherworld, shedding tears in vain. How sad! The whole world is muddled and no one is cognizant of the problem, and to not show regard for one's life, thereby treating lightly life – what eminence and influence is there to speak of?

(*continued*)

	Passage	Translation
B	而進不能愛人知人, 退不能愛身知已	Yet they are unable to care about or know others in advancing themselves in public life, and are incapable of caring about or knowing themselves in retirement.
L	遇災值禍。	They encounter disasters and face calamities.
D	身居厄地, 蒙蒙昧昧, 惷若游魂。哀乎。	They reside in a disastrous territory, and yet they remain ignorant and stupid to the point of acting like zombies. How lamentable this is!
M	趨世之士, 馳競浮華, 不固根本,	The gentlemen who flee the age still vie in their flashiness and do not fix themselves with the foundational,
N	忘軀徇物, 危若冰谷, 至於是也。	all the while disregarding their bodies as they are besotted by things. The situation has gotten to the point of being as dangerous as [treading on] ice and [facing] a ravine.
O	余宗族素多, 向余二百, 建安紀年以來, 猶未十稔, 其死亡者, 三分有二, 傷寒十居其七。感往昔之淪喪, 傷橫夭之莫救, 乃勤求古訓, 博采眾方	My clan was originally many in number, numbering in the area of more than two hundred people. Since the Jian'an reign period (196–220), it has not been ten years, and yet those who have died represent two-thirds. Of those, the number stricken from cold damage amount to seven out of ten. Moved by those who have withered to death in the past and pained by those who could not be rescued from their untimely deaths, I have exerted myself in seeking the teachings of the ancients, selecting widely from the multitudes of formulas.
S	撰用素問、九卷、八十一難、陰陽大論、胎臚藥錄, 并平脈辨證,	Consequently, I have selected from the *Basic Questions*, the *Nine Chapters*, the *Eighty-One Difficulties*, the *Great Treatise of the Yin and Yang*, the *Record of the Medicine for the Developing Fetus and Head*, as well as the [techniques] for differentiating the pulse and indicators.
P	為傷寒雜病論合十六卷, 雖未能盡愈諸病, 庶可以見病知源, 若能尋余所集, 思過半矣。	All these have been used to make the *Treatise on Cold Damage Disorders and the Miscellaneous Illnesses*, a text that altogether amounts to sixteen rolls. Although the resultant work cannot cure all illnesses, it can probably be used to apprehend the illness and understand its cause. If one is able to use what I have collected, then they will know more than most.

	Passage	Translation
F	夫天布五行。以運萬類。人稟五常,以有為五藏。經絡府俞。陰陽會通。玄冥幽微。變化難極。	Now Heaven divides into the five phases so as to move the myriad things. Man has been endowed with the five principles and so contains the five viscera, the vessels and conduits, the *qi*-repositories and transporters. The conjoining of the *yin* and the *yang* and the transformations of the dark and invisible are difficult to exhaust.
G_1	自非才高識妙,豈能探其理致哉!	If one's talent is not lofty or knowledge subtle, how could one investigate its underlying rationale and essentials!
Q	上古有神農、黃帝、岐伯、伯高、雷公、少俞、少師、仲文,中世有長桑、扁鵲,漢有公乘陽慶及倉公,下此以往,未之聞也	In high antiquity there were the Divine Husbandman, the Yellow Emperor, Qibo, Bogao, Lord Thunder, Shaoyu, Shaoshi, and Zhongwen. In the middle age, there was Changsang and Bian Que. In the Han, there was Yang Qing, of the *gongcheng* order of nobility, and the Granary Master. As for those who have come after, they have yet to be so famous.
H	觀今之醫。不念思求經旨。以演其所知。各承家伎。始終循舊。省疾問病。務在口給。相對斯須。便處湯藥。按寸不及尺。握手不及足。人迎趺陽。三部不參。動數發息,不滿五十。短期未知決診。九候曾無髣髴。明堂闕庭。盡不見察	If we consider the case of the healers of the present, they do not focus on the essential meanings of the classics or expand their knowledge. Instead, they have each inherited the techniques of their households and follow such traditions from beginning to end. In meditating on an illness and inquiring about an ailment, they are always nimble of speech, when awaiting the patient, they present a decoction or medicine promptly. In examining the pulse, they follow the inch opening but do not examine the foot, and they only press the hand. As for the feet, the [radial along with the] carotid, and the anterior tibial pulses, they do not examine these three parts. In examining the breath and pulse, they do not wait for fifty pulsations or exhalations. In cases of death, they do not know how to conduct examinations or make determinations, and it was as if the nine indicators left no impression on them. They do not look at or examine the nose, brows, or forehead.
I	所謂窺管而已。夫欲視死別生,實為難矣。	This is what is called looking through a bamboo tube (e.g., having a constricted view). If one desires to perceive impending death and pick out the patients who will live, it would be difficult [under these conditions].

(*continued*)

	Passage	Translation
R	孔子云: 生而知之者上, 學則亞之, 多聞博淺, 知之次也。余宿尚方術, 請事斯語	Confucius had said, "Those born knowing are in the highest class; those who know through learning are secondary, and those who know through persistent inquiry and broad experience follow last." I have prized the formulas and techniques, and so allow me to follow through with these words.

NOTES

INTRODUCTION

1 Needham and Lu 2000: 42–3; 45.
2 Ibid., 51.
3 Lu and Needham 1980: 117.
4 Ibid., 117.
5 Needham and Lu 2000: 52.
6 Sivin 2007: xv.
7 Fan Xingzhun 1986. For the emphasis on the achievements of medical founders, see Chen Bangxian 1937, Chen Cunren 1968; Liu Boji 1974; Ma Boying 1994; Zhu Jianping 2003. For similar examples in English, see Lee T'ao 1953; Wong K. Chimin [Wang Jimin] and Wu Lien-teh 1932.
8 On the mythical character of Bian Que, see Han Jianping 2007; Lo 2013: 33.
9 Harper 2001; Hsu 2010; Li Jianmin 2000; Sivin 1995; Yamada 1998; Yamada 2003: 413–38.
10 Liao Yuqun 2011.
11 http://www.nlm.nih.gov/exhibition/chinesemedicine/emperors.html.
12 Jin Shiqi 2010: 211–89.
13 Trautmann 1997: 19.
14 Jensen 1997; for the construction of caste, see Dirks 2001; for world religions, see Masuzawa 2005. Also see in this same vein, Sun 2013.
15 Clunas 1997.
16 Jensen 1997. For a reading of early Chinese sources that builds upon Jensen, see Denecke 2010. For critical reflections on Chinese philosophy, see DeFoort 2001a.
17 On this point, see Jensen 1997: 5, 65, 71, 119–21. Some parts of Jensen's arguments are critically analyzed and elaborated in Standaert 1999.
18 For my criticism of interpretations of Attendant He, see Brown 2012. For an older view of the Hippocratics, see Temkin 1991: 190. For more nuanced understandings of the relationship between the Hippocratics and religious healing, see Lloyd 2004: 40–83; Nutton 2004: 103-14.

19 See Low 1998. For Needham's positivism, Hart 1999; Hinrichs 1998; Sivin 2000: 16. On Needham's evolutionism, see Brown 2006: 237–42.

20 Trautmann 2011: 16.

21 This criticism is a commonplace one; for a notable example, see Eaton 2000.

22 This fact is remarked upon by Jensen but its significance is left unelaborated. On this point, see Jensen 1997: 60. Ricci's collaboration with Xu Guangqi 徐光啟 (1562–1633) is treated at length by Hsia 2010. For James Legge's close ties to his Chinese collaborator and his "slavish reliance" on the classical commentaries of Zhu Xi 朱熹 (1130–1200), see Giradot 2002: 9, 60–1. For the role that indigenous scholars played in Benjamin Hobson's translation of Western medical ideas in the mid-nineteenth century, see Andrews 1997: 122. For collaboration between indigenous and Western naturalists, also see Mueggler 2011.

23 A number of works outside of the China field have argued that Orientalist and religion scholars were influenced by indigenous intellectual traditions and movements. For Southeast Asia, see Blackburn 2001; Hallisey 1995. Some historians of India emphasize the influence of premodern Indian systems of knowledge on modern scholarship. For arguments concerning the connections between modern linguistics and Indian theories of grammar, see Trautmann 2006. Also see Wagoner 2003; and Peabody 2001.

24 For the legacies of the Qing tradition of evidential learning in contemporary China, see Pollack 2009: 944–5.

25 Denecke 2010: 33–4, 54, 61.

26 Csikszentmihalyi 2002.

27 Zheng Jinsheng and Li Jianmin 1997.

28 This is a statement that I have drawn from the appendices in Liu 1995: 274–5. Liu shows us that *yixue* 醫學 is a neologism that was used originally by seventeenth-century missionaries to translate "the study of medicine." *Yixue* later comes to mean "medicine" through the Japanese neologism *igaku*.

29 Wu Yiyi 1994: 37.

30 Duan Yishan et al. 1986: "Jiayi jing xu 甲乙經序," 229; Huangfu Mi, *Zhenjiu jiayi jing jiaozhu*, "xu 序," 16–24.

31 For a loose use of the term *bricolage*, one that overlooks the contrast between the engineer and the *bricoleur*, see Steven Shapin's discussion of Boyle's public persona in Shapin 2010: 142–3; 181.

32 Furth 1999: 14–15.

33 Lévi-Strauss 1966: 17–20.

34 Lo 2013; Hinrichs 2013a.

35 Li Jianmin 2000: 84.

36 Sivin 1995: 195; Lloyd and Sivin 2002: 23–5; Sivin 2012: 223–4. Sivin's understanding of professions draws from the influential formulation in Freidson 1970.

37 Sivin 2012: 224.

38 *Liji jijie*, "Wangzhi" 王制, 13.368. Also see the proclamation in a dynastic history that calls for healers (*yi*), merchants, and invocators to be registered with the state. On this point, see Ban Gu, *Hanshu*, 24B.1181; Jin Shiqi 2005: 25.
39 On the heterogeneity of middle-period practitioners referred to as *yi*, see Fan Jiawei 2010a: 334. Also see Hymes 1987: 13n10.
40 See the case of Liu Zu 劉租 in Chen Shou, *Sanguo zhi*, 29.800.
41 See for example references to *yaoyigong* 藥醫工 in unpublished administrative strips from the Northwest in Xie Guihua 2005: 98.
42 See the case of Chunyu Yan 淳于衍 (91–41 BC), who was referred to as *ruyi* 乳醫 (attendant for nurses) in Ban Gu, *Hanshu*, 68.2952; and Yi Xu 義姁 (fl. 109 BC), who is said to have "attended" (醫 *yi*) the Empress Dowager Wang during her illness. On this point, see Ban Gu, *Hanshu*, 90.3652; Sima Qian, *Shiji*, 122.3144.

1 ATTENDANT HE: INNOVATOR OR PERSONA?

1 I will refer to Yi He 醫和 as "Attendant He" rather than "Physician He" throughout this chapter. This decision owes something to the indefinite scope of *yi* in preimperial texts, a point discussed in Chapter 4. Because our sources imply that Attendant He was someone with a facility for diagnosing and treating ills, I will refer to him as a practitioner of the healing arts or healer throughout.
2 Zhu Jianping 2003: 63.
3 For a recent iteration of this view, see Wang Aihe 2000: 102–3. Also see Cook 2013. Cook is agnostic about Attendant He's historicity (she mentions that the story about him in the *Tradition of Zuo* is suspected by some to be a post–300 BC addition). However, she affirms the received view of him refuting "the traditional diagnosis of a spiritual curse or demonic influence." Also see Yao Chunpeng 2008: 5; Lu and Needham 1980: 144.
4 Yamada 1988: 77–9.
5 Kuriyama 1999: 252.
6 Schaberg 2001: 8–11; Egan 1977: 339–40, 348; Li Wai-yee 2007: 47–59. For a different view of the dating of the *Tradition of Zuo*, see Pines 2002: 13–54; 233–46.
7 Schaberg 2001: 26–7.
8 *Zuozhuan zhushu* [Zhao 1], 41/10b–13b; *Chunqiu Zuozhuan zhu*, 1217–21.
9 *Zuozhuan zhushu* [Zhao 1], 41/13b; *Chunqiu Zuozhuan zhu*, 1221.
10 I am following the emendation of the eminent scholar Wang Niansun 王念孫 (1744–1832) of the eight-character line (*shi wei jin nü shi, ji ru gu* 是謂近女室,疾如蠱). Wang argues that *shi* 室 (quarters) is a graphic error for *sheng* 生 (to generate, produce). The line thus should read as two four-character lines: *shi wei jin nü, sheng ji ru gu* 是謂近女, 生疾如蠱. In addition, the

term *gu* is notoriously difficult to translate, with scholars rendering the term differently and translating it as "bewitchment" or "infestations of bugs." For the former, see Kalinowski 2009: 359. For the latter, see Harper 1998: 74–5. Also see Jiang Dianwei 2003; Smith 1989: 428–30; 444–5; Xing Wen 2013.

11 *Zuozhuan zhushu* [Zhao 1], 41/13b–15b; *Chunqiu Zuozhuan zhu,* 1221–3; Li Wai-yee 2007: 132–3.

12 The passage has sparked considerable debate about its exact interpretation. Du Yu 杜預 (AD 222–84) has interpreted the passage as such: "Women usually attend to men, and thus this [intercourse] is referred to as *yangwu*" (*nü chang sui nan, gu yan yangwu* 女常隨男,故言陽物). Kong Yingda 孔穎達 (574–648), in contrast, says: "Because women are used for intercourse, the body of the lord thus became heated; and since intercourse occurs during periods of darkness, the lord has thus suffered from avolition and *gu*" (*yi nü yangwu, gu nei re, yi huishi, gu huo gu ye* 以女陽物,故內熱;以晦時,故惑蠱也). See *Chunqiu Zuozhuan zhushu*, 41/15a. The term *wu* has been glossed by Yang Bojun (*Chunqiu Zuozhuan zhu,* 1222) as referring to "serving" (*shi* 事), and so the passage would read, "With respect to women, they attend to intercourse during periods of darkness." Li Wai-yee 2007: 147 interprets the passage somewhat differently, reading the passage as follows: "As the female brings out the *yang* in things and belongs to the hours of darkness; excessive intimacy with them breeds the sickness of inner heat, confusion, and spells."

13 *Zuozhuan zhushu* [Zhao 1], 41/14a–15a; *Chunqiu Zuozhuan zhu,* 1222.

14 *Zuozhuan zhushu* [Zhao 1], 41/13b.

15 Lai Guolong 2005: 11.

16 Kalinowski 2009: 384.

17 See *Chudi chutu Zhanguo jiance (shisizhong),* 94–5 (Baoshan strips no. 218–19; 221–2, 237, 239–41); also see Cook 2006: 178–9, 182, 198–9, 200–1.

18 *Zuozhuan zhushu* [Zhao 1], 41/13b.

19 Ibid.; *Chunqiu Zuozhuan zhu,* 1221.

20 For earlier examples of *tianming* 天命 as "Heaven's will or intent," see *Shangshu* in *Duanju Shisanjing jingwen,* "Shangshu" 商書, "Pan Geng shang" 盤庚上, 13; *Chuci buzhu,* "Tian wen 天問," 3.111.

21 *Zuozhuan zhushu* [Zhao 1], 41/15a; *Chunqiu Zuozhuan zhu,* 1222–3.

22 See, e.g., *Chudi chutu Zhanguo jiance (shisizhong),* 95 (Baoshan strips no. 234–5).

23 *Zuozhuan zhushu* [Zhao 1], 41/15a–15b; *Chunqiu Zuozhuan zhu,* 1223.

24 Jin Shiqi 2009: 33–5.

25 There has been considerable debate about whether the discussion of music is metaphorical. Some traditional commentators have taken this position, but more recent interpreters have resisted this reading. See Du Zhengsheng 1995; Jin Shiqi 2009: 29.

26 *Zuozhuan zhushu* [Wen 18], 20/6a; *Chunqiu Zuozhuan zhu,* 629.

27 *Zuozhuan zhushu* [Cheng 10], 26/15a–b; *Chunqiu Zuozhuan zhu,* 849–50.

28 Li Wai-yee 2007: 240–2.

29 On the use of predictive speeches for the purposes of narrative intensification within the *Zuozhuan*, see Kalinowski 1999: 49–50.

30 Zhou Lisheng and Wang Demin 1989: 172–7.

31 Wang Aihe 2000: 102–3. Though he does not comment specifically on this incident, Marc Kalinowski offers his reflections on instances where a wise man contests the diviner's proposal to offer rites of elimination. According to Kalinowski, such contestations owe much to the general tendency in the *Tradition of Zuo* to "depreciate sacrificial and magico-religious practices" and reflect a "deep crisis of belief in the traditional techniques of divination by turtle and yarrow." For this view, see Kalinowski 2009: 372, 391, 394–5.

32 *Zuozhuan zhushu* [Zhao 1], 41/12b–13b; *Chunqiu Zuozhuan zhu,* 1220.

33 Li Wai-yee 2007: 201–2.

34 *Lunyu zhengyi,* 11/12, 449.

35 *Zuozhuan zhushu* [Zhao 1], 41/10b–12a; *Chunqiu Zuozhuan zhu,* 1217–19.

36 Li Wai-yee 2007: 238; *Zuozhuan zhushu* [Zhao 7], 44/6b–7a; *Chunqiu Zuozhuan zhu,* 1291–2.

37 *Zuozhuan zhushu* [Zhao 7], 44/5b–6a; *Chunqiu Zuozhuan zhu,* 1289–90; Li Wai-yee 2007: 237–8.

38 Kalinowski 2009: 369–73, 390.

39 For another case, see *Zuozhuan zhushu* [Xiang 10], 31/3b–4a; *Chunqiu Zuozhuan zhu,* 977.

40 *Zuozhuan zhushu* [Ai 6], 58/2a–b; *Chunqiu Zuozhuan zhu,* 1636; for another story regarding King Zhao and medical divinations, see *Chunqiu Zuozhuan* [Ai 6], 58/2a; *Chunqiu Zuozhuan zhu,* 1635–6. I follow Du Yu in interpreting the reference to "sacrifices by the great lords to the distant [gods and spirits of] the mountains, rivers, and stars within the borders" [*zhuhou wang si jingnei shanchuan xingchen* 諸侯望祀境内山川星辰]; see *Chunqiu Zuozhuan jiaozhu,* ed. Chen Shuguo ed., 1254. For a different reading, see Kalinowski 2009: 354.

41 For the first version of the episode, see *Zuozhuan zhushu* [Zhao 20], 49/5b–7b; *Chunqiu Zuozhuan zhu,* 1415–18; *Yanzi chunqiu* [*wai*], 7/3b–4b. For a second episode, see *Yanzi Chunqiu* [*nei*], 1/7b–8a; *Shanghai bowuguan cang Zhanguo Chu zhushu,* 6.159–91.

42 *Yanzi Chunqiu* [*nei*], 1/7b–8a.

43 My understanding of the manuscript draws upon the reconstruction of the text by Lai Guolong 2011a. For previous discussions, see Shen Pei 2007; Kalinowski 2009: 392–3.

44 The transcription of the text appears in Ma Chengyuan et al., *Shanghai bowuguan cang Zhanguo Chujian zhushu,* 4.195–215.

45 Schaberg 2001: 5, 17. Some differences of opinion exist as to the dates of the *Guoyu*, with estimates ranging between the fourth and second centuries BC. Yuri Pines (2002: 41–4, 262n106) treats the text as later than the *Zuozhuan*, with a mid- to late-Warring States date.

46 *Guoyu* [Jinyu 8], 14/9b–10b.

47 For representative examples, see Zhang Gao and Yu Bian, *Yi shuo,* 1/6a–6b. The *Yibu quanlu* 醫部全錄 provides quotations from Attendant He in famous Ming and Qing medical works; see Chen Menglei et al., ed., *Yibu quanlu,* 118/631; 281/1417; 340/1928. Also see Xu Chunfu, *Gujin yitong daquan,* 1/ 4. Also see Scheid 2007: 161, 171; also see the Preface of Shao Jinhan 邵晉涵 (1743–96) in Okanishi Tameto, *Song yiqian yiji kao,* 1178.

48 Li Lian, *Yi shi,* 1/223.

49 Tuotuo, *Songshi,* 255/462.13524.

2 BIAN QUE AS A SEER: POLITICAL PERSUADERS AND THE MEDICAL IMAGINATION

1 *Han Fei zi jijie*, 7/21.161.For a thorough discussion of different stories about Bian Que in the broader pre-Qin and early imperial corpus, see Liu Renyuan, Han Lijun, and Wu Chenggui 2002: 3–14.

2 Lu and Needham 1980: 85–8.

3 Yamada 2003: 351.

4 Sima Qian, *Shiji*, 105.2785;Yamada 1990: 170–8.

5 Liao Yuqun 2011: 94;Yamada 2003: 371–4; Kuriyama 1999: 162–5, 178; Li Jingwei 2007: 37–8.

6 Yamada 2003: 371. For a similar point, see Liu Renyuan, Han Lijun, and Wu Chenggui 2002: 15, 117.

7 Han Jianping 2007.

8 For a summary of most of these finds, see Li Jianmin 2000: 7–12.

9 Lewis 1999: 604.

10 Lloyd 2010; Lloyd and Sivin 2002: 27–42.

11 Sima Qian, *Shiji*, 70/63.2146–2155.

12 A parallel of one of the other episodes is found in the *Shuoyuan jinzhu jinyi*, 18/644–5. The *Shuoyuan* postdates the *Records of the Grand Historian* and so it is impossible to date this other story. At the same time, it is worth mentioning that Liu Xiang drew upon earlier works from the larger corpus of the persuaders.

13 Sima Qian, *Shiji*, 105.2786–77. In Sima's biography, Bian Que was summoned to the Jin court to revive a sick nobleman, who had assumed the leadership of the state before falling into a trance. Worried about the consequences of this turn of events, the other Jin noblemen summoned Bian Que. In a move that recalled Zichan's visit to Jin, Bian Que ruled *out* the possibility that the man's illness was due to bodily imbalance. "The blood and pulse," Bian Que told the others, "are regulated." Instead, the man's trance should be thought of as the result of divine interference: the nobleman was communing with divine beings, who were at that moment revealing the future of the Jin state. Once the gods were done, the nobleman would awake and have "things to

say." Predictably, everything was as Bian Que had predicted: the man awoke some days later with no obvious signs of illness and reported an extraordinary meeting with the gods. This story represents an obvious play on the motif of the contested divination found in the *Tradition of Zuo*. Whereas in earlier chronicles, the noble expert ruled out the influence of the spirits, in this case, a famed healer excluded bodily dysfunction as the root of the nobleman's apparent illness. Bian Que's prognosis thus represented an inversion of the leitmotif of the contested divination. In addition, such a move revealed that the author exploited the reader's expectations to provide a twist on a familiar trope – a sign, furthermore, that he was not only acquainted with but also writing within the norms of an established genre: the historical chronicle.

14 Peng Jinhua 1999. The transcriptions are found in *Guanju Qin Han mu jiandu*, 126–37. For an English-language discussion of the Guanju manuscript, see Harper 2010: 56–64.

15 *Guanju Qin Han mu jiandu*, 129.

16 For a transcription of the Mawangdui manuscripts, see *Mawangdui Han mu boshu*. For transcription and annotations, see *Mawangdui gu yishu kaoshi*. For a translation and description of its contents, see Harper 1998. A transcription of the Zhangjiashan strips can be found in *Zhangjiashan Han mu zhujian*. A corrected transcription was republished by Cultural Relics Press (Wenwu) by the same title; hereafter I will cite the 2006 edition. A study and complete translation of the Zhangjiashan *Maishu* and *Yinshu* has been done by Lo 1998 (pagination based on e-copy); for the latter work, see Lo 2014.

17 *Mawangdui gu yishu kaoshi*, 8; Liao Yuqun 1996: 2; Harper 1998: 4.

18 *Mawangdui Hanmu boshu*, 55; *Mawangdui gu yishu*, 516–17; Harper 1998: 273.

19 The first transcription of the Wuwei Hantanpo 旱灘坡 manuscript along with photographs of the original strips can be found in *Wuwei Handai yi jian*. A corrected transcription in simplified characters with annotations is found in *Wuwei Handai yijian zhujie*. Yamada Keiji provides his transcription and notes in traditional characters in Yamada 1985: 363–404. As Yamada's is still the only transcription in traditional characters, I cite his transcriptions henceforth. A transcription of medical fragments found in the northwest follows the aforementioned section of Yamada 1985: 405–15. A full site report has never been published, so the tomb number is unknown. For the report, see Gansusheng bowuguan and Gansusheng Wuweixian wenhuaguan 1973; Ma Jixing 2005: 11–12. The manuscript clearly dates to the early Eastern Han, as it contains references to General Geng Yan 耿弇 (3–58 AD); see strips 84a–84b (Yamada 1985: 394–5). For corroboration, see Chen Zhi 1988: 301; Yamada 1985: 363.

20 For coughs, see strips 3–5 (Yamada 1985: 364); for retentions, see strips 9–10 (Yamada 1985: 367); for accumulations, strips 44–45 (Yamada 1985: 379); for internal coldness, strips 48–9 (Yamada 1985: 381); for impotence and swollen scrotums, see strips 84a–84b (Yamada 1985: 394–5).

21 For theories regarding the locations of various emotional processes in medical texts, see Dong Muda 2007: 242–9.
22 *Zhangjiashan Hanmu zhujian*, 122; *Mawangdui Hanmo boshu*, 12; *Mawangdui gu yishu*, 259; cf. Harper 1998: 210.
23 Lo 1998: 80.
24 Li Bocong 1990: 68.
25 Petersen 1995: 17–19.
26 Specialist readers may wonder why I did not include several anecdotes from the biography of the Granary Master in my discussion. There are several reasons for this. As I will argue in Chapter 3, one should not assume that the biography of the Granary Master was written to serve as a guide to diagnosis or treatment like the recovered formula books and manuals for diagnosing illnesses in the vessels. That said, there are admittedly two cases (#12, 15) in which the Granary Master diagnosed an illness of which the patient was not aware: see Sima Qian, *Shiji*, 105.2805–6; 2806–7. One of these cases, however, is quite late; Elisabeth Hsu argues that the story could not have occurred before 164 BC based on the identification of personages featured in the case. See Hsu 2010: 53; Loewe 1997: 309. The remaining story may date to the earlier part of the second century. But that story does not supply evidence that healers believed that it was possible to treat illnesses before the onset of obvious symptoms. The story related the Granary Master's visit to the household of a chancellor when he spotted a slave. Noticing the slave's greenish hue, the Granary Master informed the eunuch in charge of the harem that the slave was suffering from a spleen disorder. The eunuch duly informed the chancellor, who then questioned the slave. Much like Lord Huan, the slave denied being ill ("I feel no pain"). When spring arrived, however, the slave began to feel ill and died not long afterward. Granted, the biography claimed that illnesses might be diagnosed before the onset of *discomfort*. Yet the slave's illness was obvious enough – a greenish hue is surely a sign of something amiss. Unlike Bian Que, the Granary Master never insisted upon the necessity of early treatment, nor did he indicate that it was possible to treat ills before the onset of obvious symptoms.
27 Following Ma Jixing, *Mawangdui gu yishu* (298n2) in reading *gan* 骭 as *jing* 脛.
28 *Zhangjiashan Hanmu zhujian*, 126; *Mawangdui Hanmu boshu*, 17; *Mawangdui gu yishu*, 295–8; cf. Harper 1998: 216–17.
29 For the focus in some parts of the *Maishu* on the subjective experience of pain over clinical signs, see Lo 1998.
30 *Zhangjiashan Hanmu zhujian*, "Yin shu," 177–84.
31 Ibid., 171, 184–6.
32 Liu Zhiqing 2009.
33 Needham and Lu 2000: 41
34 *Zuozhuan zhushu* [Zhao 26], 52/2a; *Chunqiu Zuozhuan zhu*, 1471.
35 *Zhanguo ce* [Han], 28/5a–5b.

36 *Zhanguo ce* [Qin], 4/4a. Here, I follow the annotations provided by He Jianzhang in *Zhanguo ce zhushi*, 127–8.
37 *Guoyu* [*Wu yu*], 19/3a.
38 *Zuozhuan zhushu* [Ai 11.4], 58/13a; *Chunqiu Zuozhuan zhu*, 1664.
39 For a summary of Mohist chronologies, see Brown 2013: 150.
40 *Mozi jiangu*, 48.418.
41 *Shizi*, ed. "Cunyi" 存疑, 67; *Shuoyuan jinzhu jinyi*, 13/429. The text of the *Shizi* was reconstructed in the Qing dynasty, and so there are questions surrounding the dates of the story from the *Shizi*. On this point, see Fischer 2009: 2–3. For another discussion of the *Shizi*, see DeFoort 2001b: 220–1.
42 Yamada 2003: 369. For an early reference to prophylaxis in politics, see Sanft 2005a: 111–12.
43 *Han Fei zi jijie*, 22/179.
44 For early texts that associate sages with wisdom, see Chen Ning 2000: 414–15; Csikszentmihalyi 2004: 169–70, 176.
45 Kalinowski 2010: 343. Also see Kalinowski 1999: 53–6. Also see in the same volume, Levi 1999: 70–3.
46 Wang Chong, *Lunheng jiaoshi*, 26/78.1075.
47 Brown and Bergeton 2008: 652–4.
48 Ibid., 649–57.
49 *Lüshi chunqiu jiaoshi*, 18/1156–7.
50 Ibid., 18/1157.
51 Knechtges 1993: 137–8; DeFoort 1997: 30, 71–99. Knechtges argues that portions of the text predate the Former Han.
52 *Heguanzi*, *xia*, 11a–11b; *Heguanzi huijiao jizhu: fu tong jian*, 335–40; 338–9.
53 Sima Qian, *Shiji*, 105.2785.
54 Yamada 2003: 351.
55 *Han Fei zi jijie*, 7/21. 161.
56 Sima Qian, *Shiji*, 105.2793–4.
57 Jin Shiqi 2010: 92; 214, 228, 261, 271–3.
58 Also see Huangfu Mi, *Huangdi zhenjiu jiayi jing*, 1/41; 5/883; Zhang Ji, *Jinkui yaolüe*, 1/17; see, e.g., *Nanjing benyi xinjie* (#77), 312; Unschuld, 1986: 630.
59 *Chongguang buzhu Huangdi neijing suwen*, 8/26.7b. The dating of the *Yellow Emperor's Inner Classic* represents a point of dispute. Three different redactions survive: the *Basic Questions* (*Suwen* 素問), the *Great Simplicity* (*Taisu* 太素), and the *Divine Pivot* (*Lingshu* 靈樞). In particular, scholarly opinion divides over the dates of the *Basic Questions*. Although some scholars have argued that the final compilation of the text was in the late first century BC or early first century AD, others have argued that the text only reached its final form in the Tang dynasty (AD 618–907), when it was arranged and commented upon by Wang Bing 王冰. For an overview of the controversies surrounding the date of the *Suwen*, see Keegan 1988; Sivin 1993. Several *pian*, namely 9, 66–71, and 74 (which treat "phase energetics") are widely regarded as

later in date, having been added by Wang Bing (see Sivin 1993: 199). For an alternative discussion of the *Huangdi neijing*, one that maintains that the *Taisu* redaction is the closest to the "original form," see Unschuld 2003: 22–58.

60 *Huangdi suwen lingshu jing*, 2/4.20a.

61 *Chongguang buzhu Huangdi neijing suwen*, 4/13.4b; 8/26.7a–b.

62 *Huangdi suwen lingshu jing*, 11/73.3a.

63 *Chongguang buzhu Huangdi neijing suwen*, 8/26.7b.

64 Ibid., 1/2.14b. For the hidden nature of many illnesses, see Kuriyama 1999: 179.

65 Zhu Danxi, *Danxi xinfa*, 2; Duan Yishan 1986, "Buzhi yibing zhi weibing lun," 177.

66 Lévi-Strauss 1962: 89.

3 CHUNYU YI: CAN THE HEALER SPEAK?

1 Historians have long noticed the inconsistent dates given for the year of Chunyu Yi's arrest. The biography of the Granary Master lists the arrest as occurring in 176 BC, whereas the *Annals of Emperor Wen* and other sources give the earlier date of 167 BC. Michael Loewe sides with the latter, citing other sources that corroborate the *Annals*. Scholars have wondered whether there is a scribal error in the former.For previous discussion of the date of Chunyu's arrest and amnesty, see Hsu 2010: 50; Loewe 1997: 305; Sanft 2005b: 81;Takigawa Kametarō, *Shiki kaichū kōshō fu kōho*, 105.20. For the earliest translation and discussion of the biography of the Granary Master into a Western language, see Bridgman 1955.

2 Sima Qian, *Shiji*, 105.2795–6.

3 Lu and Needham 1980: 106–7. For similar views, also see Chen Bangxian and Yan Lingzhou 1956: 144; Fan Xingzhun 1986: 31–3; Li Jingwei 2007: 59; Raphals 1998: 174–81.

4 Hsu 2010: 4–5. For previous attempts to reconstruct the history of Chinese medicine, particularly the development of vessel theory, based on a comparison of the *Canggong liezhuan* with excavated manuscripts, see Zhou Yimou 1994: 26. Also see Yamada 1998.

5 Duan Yishan 1986: "Jiayi jing xu," 229; Huangfu Mi, "xu," *Zhenjiu jiayi jing jiaozhu*, 16.

6 For a more skeptical view of the conventional wisdom, see Sanft 2005b. Sanft argues that other factors most likely caused Emperor Wen to reform punishments involving the mutilation of the body. The incident involving Chunyu Yi represented a convenient pretext for a reform that was already under way.

7 Sima Qian, *Shiji*, 10.427; Ban Gu, *Hanshu*, 23.1097–8.

8 Sima Qian, *Shiji*, 10.427.

9 *Lienü zhuan jiaozhu*, 6/13b–14b.

10 Opinions are divided as to whether *canggong* is an actual official title. Hsu (2010: 3) treats *canggong* as such, even though the title is unattested in the received or excavated corpus. Sivin (1995: 177) regards *canggong* as a sinecure, presumably because of the lack of evidence attesting to a position *canggong*. As Sanft points out, Chunyu Yi is referred to inconsistently in the *Shiji* as the Prefect (*ling* 令) or Head (*zhang* 長) of the Great Granaries. On this, see Sanft 2005b: 81n7. The Qin site at Liye 里耶 reveals that officials charged with directing granaries went by a number of different titles, which were used loosely. On this point, see Liu Lexian 2007: 94.

11 Hsu 2010: 52.

12 Sima Qian, *Shiji*, 105.2794–95. For a previous analysis of the chapter into sections, which departs from mine, see Hsu 2010: 49–52.

13 Sima Qian, *Shiji*, 105.2796.

14 Ibid., 105.2797–2813.

15 Ibid., 105.2813–17.

16 Ibid., 105.2817.

17 For transcriptions of Qin materials, see *Shuihudi Qin mu zhujian*. For the Shuihudi materials, I have also referred to Liu Hainian and Yang Yifan 1994: 1:375–769. The Shuihudi manuscripts have been studied extensively: two sets of translations from the corpus exist; Hulsewé 1985; McLeod and Yates 1981. For the Liye finds, see *Liye Qin jian*. A transcription can be found in *Liye Qin jiandu jiaoshi*.For the Han period: a transcription of the Zhangjiashan texts can be found in *Zhangjiashan Han mu zhujian*. I also refer to *Ernian lüling yu zouyanshu: Zhangjiashan ersiqihao Han mu chutu falü wenxian shidu*. For studies and translations of two of the legal case summaries into English, see Csikszentmihalyi 2006: 29–35; Nylan 2007.For the sites in the northwest, see *Juyan Hanjian shiwen hejiao*; *Juyan xinjian: Jiaqu Houguan yu disi sui*; *Shulehe liuyu chutu Hanjian*.

18 For the site report of the Yuelu legal materials, which were published in 2013, see Chen Songchang 2009. A full transcription is found in *Yuelu shuyuan cang Qin jian*.

19 Sanft 2013: 128.

20 Sima Qian, *Shiji*, 105.2813. For previous discussions of *fa* in medical texts, see Harper 1998: 213; also see Hsu 2010: 58; Raphals 1998: 176.

21 For the rare exception, see Jin Shiqi 2010: 234. He notes that Sima Qian apparently had some choice in how he referred to Chunyu Yi. Like Ban Gu, Sima could have referred to Chunyu Yi by the customary honorific, Master Chunyu (*Chunyu gong* 淳于公). For a perfunctory description of the bureaucratic format of the records, see Hsu 2010: 51. Hsu remarks upon the similarities but emphasizes instead the differences. She writes, "The twenty-five medical case histories record the patient's name, title of office (or relationship to a noble or king), and place of residence, much in the manner of the twenty-five legal case records of 217 BCE called 'Models for Sealing and

Investigating' (*Fengzhenshi* 封診式). However, unlike the 'Models for Sealing and Investigating,' which concerned personages identified as mister or misses XY from village YZ and which were presented as hypothetical cases, Yi's medical case histories report on past events and can be read as concerning historical individuals."

22 Sima Qian, *Shiji*, 105.2812. For Hsu's translation and explanation, see Hsu 2010: 88–9.

23 Hsu 2010: 112–15.

24 For the importance of properly classifying offenses, see Brown and Sanft 2011.

25 A similar title was found at the Mawangdui site but with different contents. According to Elisabeth Hsu, all but one of the quotations from the text found in the Granary Master's records of consultation have parallels in works transmitted through the ages. On this point, see Hsu 2010: 62.

26 Sima Qian, *Shiji*, 105.2801–2.

27 For an influential discussion of the formulaic structure of the divinatory logs, see Li Ling 2000: 273–8. For the formulaic structure of the Granary Master's records, see Hsu 2010: 109.

28 *Chudi Chutu Zhanguo jiance (shibazhong)*, 95 (strips nos. 235–8). For my translation, I have consulted both Lai Guolong (personal communication) and Guo Jue (personal communication), both of whom have worked extensively with the corpus. For a different translation, see Cook 2006: 198–9.Some notes on the translation found in the figure are necessary: (1) for the time marker in the background statement, I am following Guo Jue's reconstruction of the chronology of the Baoshan materials. (2) The phrase *hengzhen* 恆貞 has been interpreted in various ways, e.g., "long-term prognosis." I follow Chen Wei 陳偉 in glossing *heng* 恆 as *shenji* 甚吉 or *jizheng ji* 極正吉; see *Chudi chutu Zhanguo jiance*, 97n6. (3) The meaning of *shuo* 說 is still murky. It appears to have been some kind of sacrifice to the gods in response to a baleful influence, and according to Liu Xinfang, it involved using many sacrificial beasts. On this term, see Liu Xinfang 2011: 256. (4) For *yudao* 與禱 as pledge sacrifice, I am following Lai Guolong's gloss. On this point, see Lai Guolong 2011b. (5) For explanations of the sacrificial beasts, see Liu Xinfang 2011: 268–78.

29 For written directions for turtle divination, see *Yinwan Hanmu jiandu jiaoli*, 84–6 (YM6D9). For dream divination, see Chen Songchang 2009: 83–5.

30 A parallel of this story is also found in *Shuoyuan jinzhu jinyi*, 644–5.

31 Sima Qian, *Shiji*, 105.2788–91.

32 Ibid., 105.2788.

33 *Zhangjiashan Hanmu zhujian* (strips nos. 75–97), 98–9. Some notes for the translation are necessary: (1) For an extensive justification of my translation of *fa* as "class," see Brown and Sanft 2011. (2) For the quotation from the statutes, the Wenwu 2006 edition of *Zhangjiashan Han mu zhujian* reads: *mou zeiren sharen* 謀賊人殺人. This appears to be a transcription error. I thus

emend the text according to *Ernian lüling yu zouyanshu*, 354–5. The line now reads: *mou zeisha ren* 謀賊殺人.

34 See, e.g., Lu and Needham (1980: 106–7) who see the response being written after court inquiries made in 154 BC; Cullen 2001: 304–5. For discussion of the pros and cons of this view, see Hsu 2010: 50–1.

35 Jin Shiqi 2010: 232. For the original passage, see Sima Qian, *Shiji*, 105.2796. Hsu dismisses the remark in a footnote as an interpolation: "However, this sentence is odd as it is not thematically embedded in context. It reads like a late interjection into a passage concerned, first, with [Chunyu] Yi's three years of apprenticeship and, then, his age after its completion." On this point, see Hsu 2010: 50n5.

36 Jin Shiqi 2010: 231–3; Loewe 1997: 307; compare with Hsu 2010: 51–61. A similar problem with the dates was discovered by Liang Yusheng 梁玉繩 (1744–1819) in his *Shiji zhiyi*, 33/1299. For discussion of this, see Jin Shiqi 2010: 232; Takigawa, *Shiki kaichū kōshō fu kōho*, 105.23–4.

37 Hsu 2010: 58.

38 For a survey of arguments regarding Sima Qian's penchant for cutting and pasting, see Klein 2010: 13–14.

39 Loewe 1997: 305–7.

40 The biography of the Granary Master provides two different renderings of the name of Chunyu Yi's master, Yang Qing 陽慶. His surname is written inconsistently as Yang 楊 or Yang 陽. For examples of the former, see Sima Qian, *Shiij*, 105.2816, where the name is written Yang Zhongqian 楊仲倩. For both accounts of Chunyu Yi's training, see Sima Qian, *Shiji*, 105.2794; 105.2815–16; Hsu 2010: 51.

41 For *shangji* 上計 or the practice of submitting annual summaries of administrative reports from the commanderies in Han times, see the commentary of Yan Shigu 顏師古 in Ban Gu, *Hanshu*, 6.164.

42 *Liye Qin jiandu jiaoshi*, 293 (strip 8-1221). For photos of the strips, see *Liye Qinjian*, 155 (strip 8-1221).

43 The text appears jumbled. I follow Yamada in emending the passage according to parallels that appear in another manuscript from the region. For the parallels, see Yamada 1985: 391n8 (strips 80A–80B).

44 Yamada 1985: 407–8 (strip no. 1). For equivalents in metric, I have followed Wu Chengluo 1957. For translations of *materia medica*, I follow Hu Shui-ying 1999.

45 For a discussion of the discovery of formulas in the northwest, see Xie Guihua 2005.

46 *Shuihudi Qinmu zhujian*, "Fengzhen shi," 156; Liu Hainian and Yang Yifan 1994: 660–1. For Han sites with similar contents, see Li Hongfu 1982. For documents with similar contents from the northwest, also see Xie Guihua 2005.

47 Xie Guihua 2005.

48 Sima Qian, *Shiji*, 105.2813.

49 *Juyan Hanjian shiwen hejiao*, 490 (293.5). By most accounts, the Benshi reign era had only four years – this is most likely an error. Also see Li Junming 2009: 56–7. For sick logs that date to Qin and were discovered outside of frontier areas, see *Liye Qin jiandu jiaoshi*, 225 (strip II 8–780); *Liye Qinjian*, 116 (strip II 8–780).

50 *Juyan xinjian: Jiaqu Houguan yu disi sui*, 483 (E.P.F. 22.80–1); Xie Guihua 2005: 95.

51 For examples, see Xie Guihua 2005: 91–5.

52 *Juyan Hanjian shiwen hejiao*, 5 (4.4B). For further examples, see Li Junming 2009: 56; Xie Guihua 2005: 91–2.

53 *Juyan Hanjian shiwen hejiao*, [49.31], 86; Xie Guihua 2005: 97.

54 Yamada 1985: 410; Xie Guihua 2005: 85; *Shule heliuyu chutu Hanjian*, 63 (strip no. 482). For references to the errors of previous healers in the Granary Master's records, see Sima Qian, *Shiji*, 105.2799; 2808–9. For references to errors of healers mentioned by name, see Sima Qian, *Shiji*, 105.2801–2; 2809–10.

55 Ban Gu et al., *Dongguan Hanji*, 8.4a.

56 *Bajia Hou Hanshu jizhu*, 3/393–4.

57 Calculating 1 *fen* to 3.48 gm for the Later Han period per Wu Chengluo 1957: 60. Wu gives the measurements in terms of *liang* 兩; one *liang* is 4 *fen*.

58 Yamada 1985: 394. This is from the Wuwei manuscript.

59 For this identification, see Yamada, 1985: 363; De Crespigny 2007: 260–2.

60 For middle-period examples of mining the Granary Master's records, see Zhou Shouzhong (fl. 1208), *Lidai mingyi mengqiu, shang*, 2a–2b.

61 Hymes 1987: 40–1.

62 Xu Shuwei, *Leizheng buji benshi fang*, 10/6b–7a. For debates about female celibacy in Song, see Furth 1999: 89–91.

63 On this point, see Klein 2010.

64 Hsiung Ping-chen 2007: 166n5.

65 See Jiang Guan (1503–65), *Mingyi lei an*, 2/47b; 7/188a; 7/208b. See, e.g., the treatment in Wang Honghan (17th century), *Gujin yishi*, 1/18a–18b. No mention is made of the memorial of Chunyu Yi's daughter or the penal reform purportedly occasioned by Chunyu Yi's arrest. Chunyu is furthermore listed by his name. His significance is illustrated through one of the twenty-five records of consultation. A similar treatment of Chunyu Yi is found in Xu Chunfu, *Gujin yitong daquan*, 99/1395, where the case of the attendant is used to illustrate the dangers of "sensual desires that do not end (*yu buke jue* 慾不可絕)." The records of consultation are cited throughout the sections drawn from medical cases in *Yibu quanlu*, 169/308. For the importance of cases for medical thinking and other forms of knowledge in imperial China, see Furth 2007.

4 LIU XIANG: THE IMPERIAL LIBRARY AND THE CREATION OF THE EXEMPLARY HEALER LIST

1 On the creation of a classical corpus, see Nylan 2009. On the reorganization of the imperial collections, see Nylan 2011: 40–5. For the political rise of lineages after the late first century BC, see Csikszentmihalyi and Nylan 2003.

2 Here, I follow most scholars who explain *zu* 卒 as a graphic error for *za* 雜. My translation of the title reflects the assessment of Ma Jixing and many others that Zhang's original text was not exclusively limited to *Cold Damage Disorders*, an assessment based on his reading of the current preface. According to Ma, the discussion of other illnesses is preserved in a text now known as the *Essentials of the Golden Casket* (*Jinkui yaolüe* 金匱要略). On this point, see Ma Jixing 1990: 110.

3 Nylan 2000: 252; Tsien 2004: 145–50.

4 Nylan 2000: 244.

5 Nylan 2011: 100.

6 On medical initiation in early China, see Sima Qian, *Shiji*, 105.2796; Sivin 1995; Yamada 2003: 413–38. On the revelatory framework of early Chinese medicine and science, see Lloyd 1996: 26, 32ff; Lloyd and Sivin 2002: 58–60.

7 *Zhangjiashan Han mu zhujian*, "Yin shu," 171; Lo 2014: 4.

8 See, e.g., *Mawangdui gu yishu kaoshi*, 867.

9 Sima Qian, *Shiji*, 105.2785.

10 Ibid., 105.2788.

11 Ibid., 105.2815–16; Sivin 1995: 184–5.

12 On the significance of chapter titles, see Jin Shiqi 2010: 240.

13 Sima Qian, *Shiji*, 105.2794.

14 Harper 1998: 60–2.

15 On this point, see Csikszentmihalyi and Nylan 2003: 72–3; Cai Liang 2011.

16 *Chongguang buzhu Huangdi neijing*, 14/2b. For a fleeting reference to the Divine Husbandman (*Shennong* 神農), see *Chongguang buzhu Huangdi neijing*, 75/1b.

17 *Chongguang buzhu Huangdi neijing*, 1/1a–8a.

18 Ibid., 5/4a.

19 For the importance of initiation, see Sivin 1995: 187; Yamada 2003: 413–38. For the problems with using the figures found in medical works for evidence of medical lineages, see Lo and Li Jianmin 2010: 384.

20 *Chongguang buzhu Huangdi neijing*, 13/2b–3a.

21 Archaeologists have recently discovered a major cache of bamboo and wood slips with medical content in a Former Han tomb in Chengdu. The tomb probably dates to the first decades of Han and contains materials with references to Bian Que. One scholar has recently published an article, mentioning a work that archaeologists call "Bi Xi's Treatise on Medicine" (*Bi Xi yilun* 敝昔醫論). Judging from an article by Qian Yuzhi, the title represents the contrivance of modern archaeologists. On this point, see Qian Yuzhi 2014.

22 *Zhangjiashan Hanmu zhujian*, "Maishu," 126; *Mawangdui gu yishu kaoshi*, 292.
23 For the last six items, see, e.g., *Chongguang buzhu Huangdi neijing suwen*, 12/1b, 12/2a–2b.
24 Xu Shen, *Shuowen jiezi zhu*, 14.750.
25 See the *Zhouli* 周禮 in *Shisan jing zhushu: fu jiaokan ji*, 5/666–67. For discussion of these references, see Zhou Yimou 1994: 56–8.
26 See the case of Chunyu Yan 淳于衍 (91–41 BC), who was referred to as *ruyi* 乳醫 (Ban Gu, *Hanshu*, 68.2952) and Yi Xu 義姁 (act. 109 BC), who "attended the sickness" (*yi*) of the Empress Dowager Wang (Sima Qian, *Shiji*, 122.3144; Ban Gu, *Hanshu*, 90.3652).
27 Sima Qian, *Shiji*, 105.2792.
28 *Chongguang buzhu Huangdi neijing suwen*, 75/1a–75/1b.
29 For previous discussion of this passage, see Hanson 2011: 31–2.
30 *Chongguang buzhu Huangdi neijing suwen*, 12/2b.
31 Duan Yishan et al. 1986: "Shanghan lun xu" 傷寒論序, 220. For a full translation of the preface, see Appendix.
32 Ibid., "Maijing xu" 脈經序, 226.
33 Ibid., "Jiayi jing xu," 229; Huangfu Mi, *Zhenjiu jiayi jing jiaozhu*, "xu," 16–17.
34 Duan Yishan et al. 1986: "Shanghan lun xu," 220.
35 Ibid., "Maijing xu," 226.
36 Following the Zhonghua shuju editors in omitting two characters *qi ta* 其他 as textual corruption. By their account, Hua Tuo's personal name Tuo was often written in middle-period texts as *ta* 他. On this point, see Huangfu Mi, *Zhenjiu jiayi jing jiaozhu*, "xu," 16, 18n18. I have also omitted the second reference to Hua Tuo, which is redundant and a sign of textual corruption.
37 Duan Yishan et al. 1986: "Jiayi jing xu," 229; Huangfu Mi, *Zhenjiu jiayi jing jiaozhu*, 16.
38 *Huainanzi*, 19/629; Chao Yuan-ling 2009: 59, 152.
39 On this point, see Fan Jiawei 2004: 7–8.
40 Duan Yishan et al. 1986: "Jiayi jing xu," 229; Huangfu Mi, *Zhenjiu jiayi jing jiaozhu*, "xu," 17; 20.
41 Sima Qian is sometimes credited with inventing the notion of authorship. However, the mode of authorship espoused by Sima Qian was popularized by Yang Xiong 揚雄 (53 BC–AD 18); on this point, see Nylan 2011: 39–40; 59–61; Taniguchi 2010.
42 On this point, see Loewe 2014.
43 Nylan 2000: 224n29, 244; Klein 2010: 436–7, 440; Hulsewé 1975: 87.
44 Nylan 2011: 39–40; 56.
45 Ibid., 22, 36, 114–16.
46 Ibid., 53.
47 On the importance of the master's explanations, see Yamada 2003: 416–17.

48 Sivin 1995: 187.
49 Yamada Keiji is the best-known proponent of this view. See Yamada (1998, 2003) for translations in English and Chinese of essays published in the 1970s and 1980s. An English translation of his earlier, influential essays was published in 1998. A version of this view, which emphasizes the importance of initiation, also appears in Lloyd 1996: 31–4; Lloyd and Sivin 2002: 58–61.
50 For challenges to older views about transmission before the first century BC, see Nylan 2009: 742. Csikszentmihalyi and Nylan (2003: 62) have questioned whether the transmission in scholastic networks could be traced continuously over multiple generations. David Elstein (2006: 142–200) argues through his analysis of the *Biography of the Literati* in the *History of Han* that pupils frequently changed teachers. For medical transmission before the first century BC, see Harper 1998: 60–5; Keegan 1988.
51 Sima Qian, *Shiji*, 105.2796; Harper 1998: 60–5.
52 Nylan 2009: 741–2.
53 For the political rise of lineages after the late first century BC, see Cai Liang 2011; Csikszentmihalyi and Nylan 2003: 93–4; Liao Boyuan 2008: 205–24; esp. 207–8. For the lack of continuous documentation of lines of filiation, see Csikszentmihalyi and Nylan 2003: 62.
54 Nylan 2000: 244.
55 Nylan 2011: 114–15.
56 Ibid., 34, 104–5, 113–14.
57 Ibid., 107.
58 Duan Yishan et al. 1986: "Maijing xu," 226.
59 Duan Yishan et al. 1986: "Jiayi jing xu," 229; Huangfu Mi, *Zhenjiu jiayi jing jiaozhu*, "xu," 20.
60 Nylan 2011: 22.
61 Liu Xiang and Liu Xin, *Qilüe bielu yiwen, qilüe yiwen*, 106–7; Ban Gu, *Hanshu*, 10/30.1778.
62 Liu Xiang and Liu Xin, *Qilüe bielu yiwen, qilüe yiwen*, 106; Ban Gu, *Hanshu*, 10/30.1776.
63 Liu Xiang and Liu Xin, *Qilüe bielu yiwen, qilüe yiwen*, 107; Ban Gu, *Hanshu*, 10/30.1780.
64 Duan Yishan et al., 1986: "Jiayi jing xu," 229; Huangfu Mi, *Zhenjiu jiayi jing jiaozhu*, "xu," 20.
65 Lee T'ao 1940: 268–9. For official sponsorship of temples of medical progenitors and exemplary healers, see Chao Yuan-ling 2009: 62–70; Shinno 2007: 119.
66 For the introduction of Indian medicine and state-sponsored medicine, see Fan Jiawei 2007 (chs. 8–9); Salguero 2009. For the rise of medical lineages, see Leung 2013: 144; Wu Yiyi 1994.

5 ZHANG JI: THE KALEIDOSCOPIC FATHER

1 Zhang Ji was also known to premodern audiences by his style, Zhongjing 仲景. For ease of reading, I will refer to Zhang Zhongjing consistently as Zhang Ji throughout the chapter.

2 Needham and Lu 2000: 52.

3 Duan Yishan et al., 1986: "Shanghan lun xu," 220. The *Cold Damage Disorders* preface is reproduced in the Sibu beiyao version of the *Cold Damage Disorders*, as well as the early-nineteenth-century annotated edition of the text by Tamba Motohiro 丹波元簡 (1755–1810). For the latter, see *Shanghan lun jiyi*, 2–5. The former cites the Song edition of 1065 as the source of the preface's contents. The edition of 1065 was reprinted in a more affordable small-character version in 1088, on which Zhao Kaimei 趙開美 based a 1599 version (now known commonly by the misleading appellation of the "Song version"). For this, see *Zhang Zhongjing quanshu*, "Shanghan zubing lunji" 傷寒卒病論集, 1a–2b. No copies of the eleventh-century version have been recovered, but a few copies of the Ming dynasty edition are stored in several libraries around the world. By Qing times, the original Song edition published in 1065 was reportedly lost. On this point, see the comments by Zhou Shengwu 周省吾 in Taki Mototane, *Zhongguo yijikao*, 24/393. Qian Chaochen has examined the different versions of the Ming dynasty edition and confirmed that Zhang Ji's preface is reproduced in Japanese and Chinese copies of the text. Copies of this Ming dynasty edition are also reproduced in the Qing dynasty compendium, *Zhongjing quanshu* 仲景全書. On this point, see Qian Chaochen 2010; Goldschmidt 2009: 101. Aside from the edition of 1088, an annotated copy of the *Cold Damage Disorders* based on the eleventh-century edition was published by the healer Cheng Wuji 成無己 (ca. 1063–1156) in 1144. For discussions of this text, see Wang Yong and Gao Ailing 2006.

4 Cheng Yingmao, *Shanghan lun houtiao bian*, "Shanghan lun xu" 傷寒論序, 2b–3a.

5 Sima Qian, *Shiji*, 130.3300. For discussion of these themes, see Durrant 1995; Klein 2010.

6 Li Jingwei 2007: 73–4, 76.

7 Liao Yuqun 2011: 96–8.

8 For other evidence of the epidemic of late Han and particularly of AD 217, see Hanson 2011: 5–6. For evidence that the preface is referring to the epidemic of AD 217, see De Crespigny 2010: 36, 420.

9 Kuhn and Brook 2009: 1.

10 On this point, see Kuhn and Brook 2009: 41–3; Tsien 1985: 159.

11 Duan Yishan et al. 1986: "Shanghan lun xu," 220. For a full translation, see Appendix.

12 For statements of the conventional wisdom, see Chen Bangxian and Yan Lingzhou 1956: 132, 139; Fan Xingzhun 1986: 43–4, 50; Li Jingwei

2007: 76; Liu Boji 1974: 67–9; Ma Boying 1994: 283–5; Ye Fazheng 1995: 20; Zhang Taiyan 1982: V: 89–91. Also see Goldschmidt 2009: 96, 145; Hanson 2011: 5–6.

13 Li Jingwei 2007: 75.

14 For summaries of questions, see Zhu Diguang 1985. For views that Zhang Zhongjing (or Zhang Ji) was one and the same as Zhang Xian 張羨, see Chen Zhi 1998: 287. The problems with this view have long been known to historians. The internal evidence of the preface suggests that it was written around AD 205, whereas Zhang Xian, whose activities were well-known because of his political importance, died in 200. On this point, see Chen Shou, *Sanguo zhi*, 6.211–12; Fan Ye, *Hou Hanshu*, 74/64B.2421.

15 Duan Yishan et al. 1986: "'Jiayi jing xu," 229; Huangfu Mi, *Zhenjiu jiayi jing*, "xu," 17.

16 Fan Jiawei 2010a: 23. References to Zhang Zhongjing appear in virtually all early works of medicine, the majority of which are in the current version of the *Waitai miyao* 外臺秘要. For this, see Wang Tao, *Waitai miyao*, Chapter 1 (on cold damage). For other examples, see Ge Hong, *Zhouhou beiji fang*, 1/3b; 1/6a; 3/45b; 4/78a; Sun Simiao, *Beiji qianjin yaofang*, "xu," 6a-6b; "xuli," 1.1a; 4.3b. Also see the Japanese edition of the *Formulas Worth a Thousand Gold*. According to the editors, the text was discovered during the Qing dynasty and produced in part on the basis of a handwritten manuscript from Tang. As such, this edition may reflect the state of the text prior to the Song edition and thus free of the interventions of the eleventh-century Song editors. For references to Zhang Ji, see Sun Simiao, *Sun Zhenren qianjin fang: fu zhenben qianjin fang*, "xu," 1.

17 *Dunhuang guyiji kaoshi*, 21, 127, 346; *Dunhuang yiyao wenxian jijiao*, 59, 183, 548–9.

18 Chao Yuanfang, *Zhubing yuanhou lun jiaozhu*, 6/177; *Zhubing yuanhou lun jiaoshi, di'er ban*, 6/119–20.

19 Chao Yuanfang, *Zhubing yuanhou lun jiaozhu*, 6/177; *Zhubing yuanhou lun jiaoshi*, 6/119–20.

20 For examples of surgical feats attributed to Zhang Zhongjing by Ge Hong, see *Baopuzi neipian jiaoshi*, 5/101.

21 For Zhang Ji's relations with his master, see the quotations from the *Separate Biography of He Yong* (*He Yong biezhuan* 何顒別傳), adduced in Li Fang et al., *Taiping yulan*, 444/2172b; 722/3328b. Zhang Ji's superiority to his master is discussed in extant fragments from a lost Tang dynasty work, the *Record of Famous Yi* (*Mingyi lu* 名醫錄) of Gan Bozong 甘伯宗 (which circulated in the eleventh century). For quotations, see Zhou Shouzhong, *Lidai mingyi mengqiu, xia*, 28a–b.

22 Sun Simiao, *Sun Zhenren Qianjin fang*, 1/2.

23 For the earliest versions of the first story, see Duan Yishan et al., 1986: "'Jiayi jing xu," 229; for the earliest version of the second (which quotes the *Separate*

Biography of He Yong), see Li Fang et al., *Taiping yulan*, 739/3480a; *Taiping guangji*, 218/1665.

24 To be sure, the corpus of materials that discuss Zhang Ji even in premodern times is immense (a search of the Four Treasuries database, e.g., yields more than three thousand references to his name). For representative views of the text before the twentieth century, I have relied heavily upon the anthologies produced by Taki Mototane (1789–1827), Okanishi 1977, and Yan Shiyun 1990. For the latter, see Yan Shiyun 1990: 207–43.

25 For the text of the preface, see *Shanghanlun banben daquan*, 61–2.

26 For the Song preface by Lin Yi and others, see *Xinji Songben shanghan lun*, 1; Okanishi 1977: 350–2.

27 For references to the epidemic, see the remarks of Chao Gongwu 晁公武 (twelfth century) in his *Junzhai dushu zhi jiaozheng*, 15/708. For quotations of this text in a Yuan dynasty biographical sketch of Zhang Ji, see Ma Duanlin (1254–1323), *Wenxian tongkao*, 222/1794a. For representative examples of similar comments in later texts, see the remarks of Fang Youzhi 方有執 (b. 1522) in the *Shanghan lun tiaobian*, "yin" 引, 1a; Li Lian, *Yi shi*, 6/2b; *Yibu quanlu*, "Yishu mingliu liezhuan" 醫術名流列傳, 505/97; Wang Honghan, *Gujin yishi*, 1/20a–b. Also see the *Yilin liezhuan* 醫林列傳 preserved in *Zhongjing quanshu*, "Liezhuan" 列傳, 1a.

28 Guo Yong, *Zhongjing shanghan bu wang lun*, "xu," 3a; Okanishi, 1977: 461.

29 See the postface by Yan Qizhi 嚴器之 (fl. 1241–52) in Cheng Wuji, *Shanghan mingli lun*, "xu," 3a; Okanishi, 1977: 327.

30 For Liu's remarks, see Liu Wansu, *Suwen xuanji yuanbing shi*, 5; Taki, *Zhongguo yiji kao*, 23/364. Also see the remarks of Yu Chang 喻昌 (1585–1664), which resonate with those of Liu; Yu Chang, *Shanglun pian*, "juan shou 卷首," 1a; Taki, *Zhongguo yiji kao*, 24/379.

31 Goldschmidt 2009: 11, 70; Ma Jixing 1990: 117–18, 121, 123.

32 Based on the references to Zhang Ji and the existence of different editions of the *Cold Damage Disorders*, Stephen Boyanton has concluded that the *Cold Damage Disorders* was not a long-neglected text, as Asaf Goldschmidt argues. Instead, the treatise was "both well-known and highly valued" in the early medieval period. However, Boyanton does acknowledge the role that the mass printing of the text played in increasing its circulation and the fact that the manuscript probably circulated in different, shorter forms than the Song version. On this point, see Boyanton (Forthcoming).

33 For remarks about the poor state of the text, see the Song postface, preserved in *Xinji Song ben Shanghan lun*, 1. For comments regarding the rearrangement of the text in the centuries after Zhang Ji's death, see Zhang Canjia 1998: 146.

34 One Dunhuang manuscript, attributed to Zhang Ji, is clearly post-Han in date, as it references figures from later centuries. For this, see *Dunhuang guyiji kaoshi*, 21; *Dunhuang yiyao wenxian jijiao*, 59; Cullen and Lo 2005: 387.

35 Goldschmidt 2009: 100–1. For Lin Yi's remarks about the *Jinkui yaolüe*, see *Zhongjing quanshu*, "Jinkui yaolüe fanglun xu," 1a; Taki, *Zhongguo yiji kao*, 25/399. Also see Ma Jixing 1990: 121.

36 Goldschmidt 2009: 45, 88, 93–4.

37 Ibid., 80–1; though in agreement about the spike of epidemics in Song, Fan Jiawei 范家偉 (Fan Ka Wai) is critical of Goldschmidt's discussion of the precise nature and origins of the epidemics. On this point, Fan Ka Wai and Sze-nga Lau, 2010: 233. A fuller version of the review by Fan also appeared in Chinese: see Fan Jiawei 2010b.

38 For an example, see the *Guqin shu* 古琴疏 of Yu Ruming 虞汝明 (Song) in Okanishi 1977: 313. I have not been able to track down Yu's original text, as the *Guqin shu* appears to be a rare book. However, the passage is also quoted by Yan Shiyun 1990: 208.

39 For the persistence of older ways of narrating Zhang Zhongjing's life beyond the eleventh century, see Zhang Gao and Yu Bian, *Yi shuo*, 1/12b; 14a; Zhou Shouzhong, *Lidai mingyi mengqiu*, *xia*, 28a–b.

40 For the origins of the term *ruyi*, see Goldschmidt 2009: 56–7.

41 Hymes 1987: 23.

42 For the example of Xu Shuwei, see Hymes 1987: 40–1. Fan Jiawei argues that Goldschmidt has exaggerated the degree to which healers were a despised group in the middle period. For this, see Fan Ka Wai and Lau Sze-nga 2010: 234.

43 Sivin (Forthcoming).

44 Hymes 1987: 37–9.

45 Compare this claim, however, with Fan Ka Wai and Lau Sze-nga (2010: 234), who document Tang imperial patronage of medicine.

46 Goldschmidt 2009: 20–1, 56–7. For cultural changes that enabled the rise of genteel healers, see Chen Yuanpeng 1997; Leung 2003.

47 On this well-known point, see Chaffee 1995; Hymes 1986.

48 Shinno highlights in particular the collaborations of the Mongols, their *semu* advisors, and Chinese elites in creating a hospitable environment for healers. On this point, see Shinno 2007: 94–5.

49 Hymes 1987: 57.

50 See the quotation from Jia Huangzhong 賈黄中 (941–90) in Zheng Qiao, *Tongzhi* 通志, 113/181.2895a, Goldschmidt 2009: 25.

51 Goldschmidt 2009: 93.

52 Li Jingwei 2007: 75.

53 See *Xinji Songben shanghan lun*, 1. Remarks in this vein are innumerable.

54 Liu Wansu, *Suwen xuanji yuanbing shi*, 5; Taki Mototane, *Zhongguo yiji kao*, 23/364; Goldschmidt 2009: 60.

55 Hanson 2003: 121; Chao Yuan-ling 2009: 44–8.

56 Goldschmidt 2009: 20–1.

57 For quotations, see Zhou Shouzhong, *Lidai mingyi mengqiu*, *xia*, 28a–b.

58 On these points, see Nylan 2009; Sivin 1995.

59 Sima Qian, *Shiji*, 110.2919.

60 *Xinji Shanghan lun*, "xu," 1.

61 Liu Wansu, *Suwen xuanji yuanbing shi*, 5–6; Okanishi 1977: 332; for Yan Qizhi, see his postface to the *Zhujie shanghan lun*, 1b; Taki, *Zhongguo yiji kao*, 23/364; for Lü Fu, see *Yibu quanlun* (502.33), which preserves an essay by Lü Fu, "Gufang lun" 古方論, from *Yimen qunjing bianlun* 醫門羣經辨論 (to the best of my knowledge, this work no longer circulates as an independent title); Taki, *Zhongguo yiji kao*, 23/365.

62 Liu Wansu, *Suwen xuanji yuanbing shi*, 5–6; Okanishi 1977: 332; also see the comments of Wu Cheng 吳澄 (1249–1333) in Wu Cheng, *Wu Wenzheng ji*, 19/6b; in Taki Mototane, *Zhongguo yiji kao*, 23/364. For similar concerns in late imperial China, see Hanson 2011: 95.

63 Chen Zhensun, *Zhizhai shulu jieti*, 814; Taki Mototane, *Zhongguo yiji kao*, 23/363.

64 Hanson 2011: 39; 124–5.

6 HUANGFU MI: FROM INNOVATOR TO TRANSMITTER

1 Porkert 1974: 201

2 Unschuld 2003: 22–4.

3 Chen Bangxian and Yan Lingzhou 1956: 96.

4 Duan Yishan et al. 1986: "Jia yi jing xu," 229.

5 Liao Yuqun 2011: 98–9. For similar efforts to cast Huangfu Mi as a book worm rather than a master healer, see Ma Boying 1994: 432–4. For similar views of Huangfu Mi, see Li Jingwei 2007: 98–100. Li devotes exactly two sentences to Huangfu Mi's experiments with mineral ingestion. Also see Chen Cunren (1968: 50–1).

6 *Lunyu zhengyi*, 7/1, 251.

7 Duan Yishan et al. 1986: "Jiayi jing xu," 229; Huangfu Mi, *Zhenjiu jiayi jing*, "xu," 20–1.

8 On this, see DeClercq 1998: 159–205.

9 Ibid., 159.

10 Ibid., 161–4.

11 Ibid., 171–2.

12 On Huangfu Mi's corpus, see Knapp 2000: 3–4; Fang Xuanling (578–648) et al. *Jinshu*, 21.1418.

13 Yu Jiaxi 1997: "Hanshi san kao" 寒食散考, 166–209; esp. 202. Yu estimated that 80 to 90 percent of Huangfu Mi's writings on the subject survive in quotations.

14 Although Chao Yuanfang has been traditionally credited with the compilation of the *Zhubing yuanhou lun*, this attribution is not without problems.

According to Fan Jiawei (2007: 51) at least another figure may have been responsible for this work.

15 For the canonical status of Huangfu Mi's *Jiayi jing*, see Fan Jiawei 2010a: 187; Fan Jiawei 2013: 89.

16 Lo and Li 2010: 396.

17 Unschuld 2003: 22–3. Scholars estimate that up to two-thirds of the present *AB Classic* comprise the *Basic Questions* and *Divine Pivot*. On this point, see Dong Fayao 2012: 37.

18 On the makeup of cold food powder, see Fan Xingzhun 1986: 52; Yu Jiaxi 1997: 173. For sources that trace the powder to the biography of the Granary Master in the *Records of the Grand Historian*, see Needham 1974: 287–8; Zhang Canjia 1998: 57. Other accounts, however, place its discovery in the late Han; on this point see, Yu Jiaxi 1997: 167–8. Also see the German-language article by Wagner 1973 (I do not read German, so I will not refer to its contents).

19 Chao Yuanfang, *Zhubing yuanhou lun*, 6/177; *Zhubing yuanhou lun jiaoshi, di'er ban*, 6/119–20.

20 Chao Yuanfang, *Zhubing yuanhou lun*, 6/177; *Zhubing yuanhou lun jiaoshi, di'er ban*, 6/120.

21 This is quoted in Li Fang et al., *Taiping yulan*, 722/3330b as the *Jinshu* of Wang Yin 王隱 (fl. 276–323); *Taiping yulan*, 743/3430b. Also see *Dunhuang guyiji kaoshi*, "Fuxing jue zangfu yongyao fayao," 127; *Dunhuang yiyao wenxian jijiao*, 183.

22 For references to titles that approximate the *Jiayi jing*, see Wei Zheng (580–643) et al., *Suishu*, 34.1040; Yong Rong (1744–90) et al., *Siku quanshu zongmu tiyao*, 103/2086. For the other works attributed to Huangfu Mi, see *Suishu*, 34.1045; 34.1041.

23 For the late date of works that attribute the *Jiayi jing* to Huangfu Mi, see DeClercq 1998: 167n30.

24 For the sole exception, see Wang Tao, *Waitai miyao*, 39/1077a. For Huangfu Mi's suicide attempt after ingesting the powder, see *Waitai miyao*, 37/1041a.

25 Epler 1977: 255–62.

26 Tanba Yasuyori, *Ishinpō*, 19/780; *Ishinpō*, tr. Maki Sachiko, 19/54; Chao Yuanfang, *Zhubing yuanhou lun jiaozhu*, 6/199; *Zhubing yuanhou lun jiaoshi, di'er ban*, 6/142.

27 Chao Yuanfang, *Zhubing yuanhou lun*, 6/177; *Zhubing yuanhou lun jiaoshi, di'er ban*, 6/120.

28 Chao Yuanfang, *Zhubing yuanhou lun jiaozhu*, 6/178; *Zhubing yuanhou lun jiaoshi, di'er ban*, 6/120.

29 Chao Yuanfang, *Zhubing yuanhou lun jiaozhu*, 6/177–8; *Zhubing yuanhou lun jiaoshi, di'er ban*, 6/119–20.

30 Chao Yuanfang, *Zhubing yuanhou lun jiaozhu*, 6/203; *Zhubing yuanhou lun jiaoshi, di'er ban*, 6/146.

31 Chao Yuanfang, *Zhubing yuanhou lun jiaozhu*, 6/178; *Zhubing yuanhou lun jiaoshi, di'er ban*, 6/120.

32 Chao Yuanfang, *Zhubing yuanlun jiaozhu*, 6/194; *Zhubing yuanhou lun jiaoshi, di'er ban*, 6/138. Also see *Taiping yulan*, 738/3403b.

33 Translation adapted from DeClercq 1998: 186; Fang Xuanling, *Jinshu*, 21.1415. I have largely amended his renderings of medical terminology like *weicuo jiedu* 違錯節度 ("to err with respect to dosage" as opposed to "acting contrary to my system"), *haini* 咳逆 ("coughing and reversal" as opposed to "phlegm obstructed my throat"), *nüe* 瘧 ("hot and cold spells" as opposed to "malaria"), and *shanghan* 傷寒 ("cold damage" as opposed to "stricken with a cold").

34 DeClercq 1998: 184.

35 Cherniack 1994: 53.

36 For the longevity of the cold food powder craze, see Fan Xingzhun 1986: 56.

37 Sun Simiao, *Beiji qianjin yaofang*, 24/433a; 1/2b. For warnings in Ge Hong, see *Zhouhou beiji fang*, 3/22.57b.

38 Tanba Yasuyori, *Ishinpō*, 19/777; *Ishinpō*, tr. Maki Sachiko, 19/24.

39 Tanba Yasuyori, *Ishinpō*, 19/775; *Ishinpō*, tr. Maki Sachiko, 19/10.

40 Tanba Yasuyori, *Ishinpō*, 19/777; *Ishinpō*, tr. Maki Sachiko, 19/24.

41 Tanba Yasuyori, *Ishinpō*, 19/777; *Ishinpō*, tr. Maki Sachiko, 19/24.

42 Tanba Yasuyori, *Ishinpō*, 2/98; *Ishinpō*, tr. Maki Sachiko, 2b/9.

43 Wang Tao, *Waitai miyao*, 39/1077a.

44 Liu Xu (887–946), *Jiu Tangshu*, 47.2046; Ouyang Xiu (1007–72) and Song Qi (998–1061), *Xin Tangshu*, 50.1565.

45 For an eleventh-century example of Huangfu Mi being presented as an expert on cold food powder, see, e.g., Wang Qinruo et al., *Cefu yuangui* of the eleventh century, 205/10193b; Okanishi 1977: 1403.

46 On the bureau's efforts to edit the text, see Unschuld 2003: 23–4.

47 Huangfu Mi, *Zhenjiu jiayi jing*, "xu," 12. For a similar observation, see Epler 1977: 267.

48 Goldschmidt 2009: 38.

49 For passages that use Huangfu Mi's remarks as evidence of the Yellow Emperor's authorship of the *Inner Classic*, see Zhang Gao and Yu Bian, *Yi shuo* 2/1a, 2/1b.

50 Zhang Gao and Yu Bian, *Yi shuo*, 9/16a–17a. For Huangfu Mi's biography, see *Yi shuo*, 1/17b–18a.

51 *Gujin yitong daquan*, 1/13–14; Wang Honghan, *Gujin yishi*, 2/2b.

52 *Yibu quanlu*, 505/109.

53 Huangfu Mi would not have been the only editor to be sidelined by the Sui cataloguers. Descriptions of Wang Xi's hand in editing Zhang Ji's treatise are quite early (they date as early as the third or fourth century AD). Yet his role in editing any of Zhang Ji's corpus, too, is omitted from the Sui

catalogue. For Wang Xi's hand in editing Zhang Ji's corpus, see the remarks of Gao Zhan 高湛 in Li Fang et al., *Taiping yulan*, 72/3329a. For the entries to Zhang Ji's work, see Wei Zheng, *Suishu*, 34.1041.For the Qing editors' remarks, see Yong Rong et al., *Siku quanshu zongmu tiyao*, 103/2086.

54 For the parallel in surviving fragments of the *Genealogical Records*, see *Yi shuo*, 2/1a. For the intent of the *Genealogical Records*, see Knapp 2000: 4, 14–15. For a translation and discussion of the essay, see DeClercq 1998: 181–205.

55 Fang Xuanling et al., *Jinshu*, 21.1414. Here, my translation, particularly of the the line *cunjing yu dushi* 存精於獨識, departs significantly from DeClercq 1998. DeClercq renders the same line, "Hua Tuo lodged his mastery in unique diagnoses."

56 Yu Jiaxi 1997: 171. A search through the Sinica database also reveals Ming references to cold food powder in pharmacopeia.

57 The first to raise questions about the authenticity of the *Basic Questions* was Chu Cheng 褚澄 (fifth century) in *Chushi yishu*, "Bianshu" 辨書, in Feng Kebin ed., *Guang baichuan xuehai: fu suoyin*, 1114a; Taki, *Zhongguo yiji kao*, 1/1. The authenticity of the *Basic Questions* was defended by the Tang minister Fan Zhongyan 范仲淹 (989–1052), *Fan Zhongyan quanji*, 2.670.

58 Cheng Hao and Cheng Yi, *Er Cheng Yishu*, 5/213; Taki, *Zhongguo yiji kao*, 1/1; Unschuld 2003: 1–2. Unschuld and Taki attribute this passage to Cheng Yi's brother, Cheng Hao 程顥 (1032–85). But this passage is listed in the *Er Cheng Yishu* as the words of Cheng Yi. Some doubt, however, exists as to the authorship of the passage. That said, a second passage (19/317) is attributed to Cheng Yi.

59 For further examples of controversy, see Unschuld 2003: 1–2. Also see Taki, *Zhongguo yiji kao*, 1/1–2.

60 Sima Guang, *Sima Guangji*, 9/1736–37; Taki, *Zhongguo yiji kao*, 1/2; Unschuld 2003: 1.

61 Huangfu Mi, *Zhenjiu jiayi jing*, "xu," 12.

62 Ibid., 20–1.

63 Huangfu Mi, *Zhenjiu jiayi jing*, "xu," 12.

64 Zhang Gao and Yu Bian, *Yi shuo*, 2/1a. The eleventh-century author, Gao Cheng 高承, made a similar appeal, based on a parallel passage in the *Genealogical Records of Emperors and Kings*; see *Shiwu jiyuan*, 7/277; Taki, *Zhongguo yiji kao*, 1/4.

65 For Lü Fu's comments, see Dai Liang (1317–83), *Jiuling shan fang ji*, 27/12b–13b; Taki, *Zhongguo yiji kao*, 1/4–5. Lü's comments were influential enough to be repeated verbatim in the Ming dynasty compendium by Yang Jizhou, *Zhenjiu dacheng*, "Zhenjiu yuanliu" 針灸源流, 3a.

66 Yu Jiaxi 1997: 166–7; for the rare historian of medicine that lingers on Huangfu Mi's work on cold food powder, see Fan Xingzhun 1986: 51, 54–6.

EPILOGUE: ANCIENT HISTORIES IN THE MODERN AGE

1 For Ming and Qing reorderings, see Hanson 2003; Hanson 2011: 126–50.

2 On this point, see Brown 2012; Scheid 2007: 307–9; Taylor 2005: 66; Zheng Jinsheng and Li Jianmin 1997.

3 Andrews 2014: 70–1.

4 Yi-Li Wu 2013: 205.

5 Andrews 2013: 225.

6 Ibid., 219.

7 Ibid., 220.

8 Lu Xun, *Selected Stories of Lu Hsun*, "Medicine," 47–57.

9 Andrews 2013: 220.

10 Ibid., 216.

11 Ibid., 218, 225.

12 For these charges, see Wu Lien-teh 1959: 565–6; Flohr 1996: 369, 371, 373. For similar themes found in the writings of other figures, see Andrews 2013: 231. On the importance of hygiene, see Lei 2009; Rogaski 2004.

13 For the proposal to ban Chinese medicine, see Andrews 2013: 225–31; Croizier 1968: 97–145.

14 Andrews 2013: 222. For attacks on Chinese medicine that highlighted the subjective and unstandardized nature of diagnosis and treatment, see Scheid 2012: 13–15.

15 Andrews 2013: 222.

16 Lei 2002: 345.

17 Andrews 2013: 234–8.

18 Ibid., 236–8.

19 On standardization, see Scheid 2002: 230. For reforms involving the transmission of Chinese medicine and the publication of secret family formulas, see Scheid 2007: 309.

20 For the hybridity of contemporary incarnations of Chinese medicine, see Mei Zhan 2009: 131–42; Scheid 2001; Scheid 2002.

21 Farquhar 1994. For efforts to tie new practices to classical texts, see Scheid 2008.

22 Scheid 2007: 382.

23 Andrews 2013: 223, 226–7; Andrews 2014: 136–41.

24 Andrews 2013: 226. For Chen's role within this movement, see Lei 2002: 346.

25 Chen Cunren 1968.

26 On Chen's relationship to Ding Fubao, see Zhao Hongjun 1989: 180. For a sketch of Ding, see Andrews 2014: 122–33.

27 For Chen's role in mentoring the first generation of medical historians in the People's Republic in the capacity as teacher and Deputy Director of the Institute of Chinese Medicine, see Zheng Jinsheng and Li Jianmin 1997: 267.

28 Lei (Forthcoming).
29 Wu Lien-teh 1959: 217.
30 Ibid., 566–7.
31 Wang Jimin 1930. On the complex attitudes of Wang and Wu toward Chinese medicine and the rationales for writing their history, see Lei (Forthcoming).
32 Chen Shou, *Sanguo zhi*, 29.799–805; for a modern translation, see DeWoskin 1983: 140–53; Ngo 1976.
33 Campany 2009: xiii.
34 Chen, *Sanguo zhi*, 29.799.
35 Ibid., 29.804.
36 Ge Hong, *Baopuzi neipian jiaoshi*, 5/101–2.
37 Zhang Gao and Yu Bian, *Yi shuo*, 1/14b; for a similar description, see Zhou Shoucheng, *Lidai mingyi mengqiu, xia*, 13a; Li Lian, *Yi shi*, 2/2a–b; *Yibu quanlu*, 505/99–100. For another description of Hua Tuo that highlights his devotion to the arts of self-cultivation, see Wang Honghan, *Gujin yitong daquan*, 1/11. This description is closely paraphrased, e.g., in the *History of Healing* of the sixteenth century and the *Biographies of Celebrated Personalities of the Arts of the Healer* (*Yishu mingliu liezhuan* 醫術名流列傳), anthologized in the *Complete Record of Healers.*
38 Wang Jimin 1930: 40. Also on this point, see the brief history by Chen Cunren 1968: 36–7; Fan Xingzhun 1986: 38–40; Liao Yuqun 2011: 96–7; Li Jingwei, 2007: 68–73; Ma Boying 1994: 289–91.
39 Wong K. Chimin and Wu Lien-teh 1932: 37.
40 Chen Cunren 1968: 36, 37.
41 Li Jingwei 2007: 72.
42 Ge Hong mentioned Hua Tuo's knowledge of techniques used for the explicit pursuit of super longevity. For this, see *Baopuzi neipian jiaoshi*, 5/102. Sun Sunmiao, for his part, offered a drug formula associated with Hua Tuo, which Sun claimed was good for forestalling aging; see Sun Simiao, *Qianjin yifang*, 12/144a. On this, see Fan Jiawei 2010a: 15–16.
43 Chen Bangxian 1937: 22.
44 Fan Xingzhun 1986: 12–13; Li Jingwei, 2007: 35–6; Ma Boying 1994: 208–9.
45 Wong K. Chimin and Wu Lien-teh 1932: 32.
46 Ibid., 35.
47 Chen Cunren 1968.
48 Ibid., 18, 20.
49 Ibid., 40.
50 Wong K. Chimin and Wu Lien-teh 1932: xvii. I have updated the romanization.
51 Biagioli 2006: 3.
52 Chen Bangxian 1937: 22; Chen Bangxian and Yan Lingzhou 1956: 237–8.
53 Wong K. Chimin and Wu Lien-teh 1932: 34–5.
54 Wagoner 2003: 784.

55 Trautmann 2006.
56 For a racy (and not necessarily comprehensive) discussion of Needham's relationship with Lu, see Winchester 2008.
57 Lu and Needham 1980: xxi.
58 Chen Bangxian and Yan Lingzhou 1956.
59 Ibid., 139. On this point, compare the sources used by Chen and Yan with those quoted in *Yibu quanlu*, 505/97.
60 Chen Bangxian and Yan Lingzhou 1956: 96.
61 Lu and Needham 1980: 328, 341.

APPENDIX: A PROBLEMATIC PREFACE

1 Wang Pinxian, Ding Qihou, Zhou Hongjin 1982. Wang and his collaborators point to two facts that undermine assumptions of Zhang's authorship: first, the preface mentioned the *Yellow Emperor's Inner Classic* as a source but did not use it; and secondly, there were references to acupoints in the preface never discussed in the *Cold Damage Disorders.* While suggestive, the arguments of Wang et al. have been largely overlooked – and justifiably so, as they are based on the faulty assumption that the extant version of the *Cold Damage Disorders* is identical to that of Han times.
2 Qian Chaochen 1993: 674–5.
3 Sun Simiao, *Beiji qianjin yaofang*, "xu," 6b; *Sun Zhenren qianjin fang*, "xu," 1.
4 *Beiji qianjin yaofang*, "xu," 6b; *Sun Zhenren qianjin fang*, "xu," 1–2.
5 *Shanghan lun banben daquan*, 61.
6 Chen Senhe and Ouyang Yu'e 2010: 36. Also see Boyanton (Forthcoming): Chapter 1.
7 One passage cites Zhang Zhongjing as his source; on this, see Sun Simiao, *Sun Zhenren qianjin fang*, "xu," 2; the other is more ambiguous and cites a work called the *Treatise on Formulas* (*Fanglun* 方論). For this, see *Sun Zhenren qianjin yaofang*, 3/5.
8 For the Japanese edition of the text, first published in 1858, see *Kangzhi ben Shanghan lun*. As Ma Jixing (1990: 134) observes, the text has notes dating to AD 805 and 1143, making it one of the earliest attested versions of the text; also see Qian Chaochen 1983. The text apparently represents a manuscript tradition that predates the Song revision of 1065.
9 On the *Formulas of Zhang Zhongjing* and its relationship to the *Cold Damage Disorders*, see Ma Jixing, who argues that the *Zhang Zhongjing fang* was one version of a text that gave rise to the present *Cold Damage Disorders*; Ma Jixing 1990: 113. Also see the remarks of Gao Zhan 高湛 in Li Fang et al., *Taiping yulan*, 722/3329a, which indicate that the *Formulas of Zhang Zhongjing* was edited by Wang Xi, a description that matches those of the *Cold Damage Disorders*.
10 Li Fang et al., *Taiping yulan*, 722/3329a.

11 Li Fang et al., *Taiping yulan*, 722/3329a.
12 For the dates, see *Shanghan lun banben daquan*, 254.
13 *Shanghan lun banben daquan*, 126–7.
14 Qian Chaochen 1993: 663–8. For the speculative theory that Kūkai 空海 (ca. fl. 805) brought the manuscript to Japan from China, see *Shanghan lun banben daquan*, 127–8.Qian Chaochen's argument hinges on two taboos. First, he argues that the Kangping edition avoids the character *jian* 堅, substituting *ying* 硬 or some variant. In his view, this is evidence of a Sui dynasty taboo. However, *jian* is found at least in one place in the text of the Kangping edition, written in small characters, which may reflect a copier attempting to add text that had been not copied in the first round. On this point, see *Shanghan lun banben*, 66. In addition, taboos were not rigorously enforced until the Song dynasty, and even then, not for private manuscripts. On this point, see Ho Pengyoke 2007: 13; Sivin 1968: 72. A similar substitution is furthermore found in much later copies, including Zhao Kaimei's edition of the *Cold Damage Disorders*, which suggests that the existence of one substitution is insufficient grounds for dating the manuscript as a whole.More important to Qian's argument is the absence of any evidence of Song taboo avoidances. On this, see Qian Chaochen 1993: 667–8; Chen Yuan 1958: 153. Qian notes that in several places, the text reads *xuan* 玄, whereas in the Zhao Kaimei edition, the same text reads *zhen* 真, which he takes as evidence of observance of a Song imperial taboo. His analysis appears to have been largely based on the main text of the *Cold Damage Disorders* and does not take into consideration the preface. True enough, we find *xuan* in the Kangping edition of the preface (see *Shanghan lun banben daquan*, 61). But we also find the same graph in the Zhao Kaimei edition, which suggests that the Song editors may not have observed the taboo. For this, see *Shanghan lun banben daquan*, 376.
15 Chen Senhe and Ouyang Yu'e 2010.
16 This passage appears in Zhang Gao and Yu Bian, *Yi shuo*, 1/14a–14b; two other passages about members of Zhang Ji's social network, cited from the *Preface to the Formulas of Zhang Zhongjing*, also appear there.
17 For the *Cold Damage Disorders* preface, see *Xinji Songben shanghan lun*, 3–4; Okanishi 1977: 350–2.

WORKS CITED

PRE-1900 WORKS

Bajia Hou Hanshu jizhu 八家後漢書輯注. Edited by Zhou Tianyou 周天游. 2 vols. Shanghai: Shanghai guji, 1986.

Ban Gu 班固 (32–92). *Hanshu* 漢書. Annotated by Yan Shigu 顏師古 (581–645). Taipei: Dingwen shuju, 1986.

Dongguan Hanji 東觀漢記. Edited by *Siku quanshu zhenben bieji* 四庫全書珍本別輯. Vols. 106–7. Taipei: Taiwan shangwu yinshuguan, 1975.

Chao Gongwu 晁公武 (12th cent). *Junzhai dushu zhi jiaozheng* 郡齋讀書志校證. 2 vols. Shanghai: Shanghai guji, 2011.

Chao Yuanfang 巢元方 (fl. 605–16). *Zhubing yuanhou lun jiaoshi, di'er ban* 諸病源候論校釋, 第二版. 2 vols. Beijing: Renmin weisheng, 2011.

Zhubing yuanhou lun jiaozhu 諸病源候論校注. Beijing: Renmin weisheng, 1991–2. Rpt. 1996.

Cheng Hao 程顥 (1032–85) and Cheng Yi 程頤 (1033–1107). *Er Cheng Yishu* 二程遺書. Edited by Pan Fu'en 潘富恩. Shanghai: Shanghai guji, 2000.

Cheng Wuji 成無己 (fl. 1063–1156). *Shanghan mingli lun* 傷寒明理論. Edited by Tao Hua 陶華. Taipei: Yiwen, 1967.

Cheng Yingmao 程應旄 (fl. 1671). *Shanghan lun houtiao bian* 傷寒論後條辨. Edited by Xuxiu Siku quanshu 續修四庫全書. Vol. 986. Shanghai: Shanghai guji, 2002.

Chen Menglei. See *Yibu quanlu*.

Chen Shou 陳壽 (233–97). *Sanguo zhi* 三國志. Annotated by Pei Songzhi 裴松之 (372–451). Taipei: Dingwen shuju, 1980.

Chen Zhensun 陳振孫 (fl. 1211–49). *Zhizhai shulu jieti* 直齋書錄解題. N.p. Guangwen shuju, 1968.

Chongguang buzhu Huangdi neijing suwen 重廣補注黃帝內經素問. Edited by Sibu congkan 四部叢刊. Part 33. Shanghai: Shangwu yinshuguan, 1937–8.

Chuci buzhu 楚辭補注. Edited by Hong Xingzu 洪興祖 and Bai Huawen 白化文. Beijing: Zhonghua shuju, 1983. Rpt. 2000.

Chudi chutu Zhanguo jiance (shisizhong) 楚地出土戰國簡册(十四種). Edited by Chen Wei 陳偉. Beijing: Jingji kexue chubanshe, 2009.

Chunqiu Zuozhuan jiaozhu 春秋左傳校注. Edited by Chen Shuguo 陳成國. 2 vols. Changsha: Yuelu shushe, 2006.

Chunqiu Zuozhuan zhu 春秋左傳注. Edited by Yang Bojun 楊伯峻. 4 vols. Beijing: Zhonghua shuju, 1990.

Dai Liang 戴良 (1317–83). *Jiuling shan fang ji* 九靈山房集. Edited by Sibu Congkan 四部叢刊. Vols. 1485–90. N.p.

Duanju Shisan jing jingwen 斷句十三經經文. Taipei: Taiwan kaiming, 1991.

Dunhuang guyiji kaoshi 敦煌古醫籍考釋. Edited by Ma Jixing 馬繼興 and Yu Wenzhong 于文忠. Nanchang: Jiangxi kexue jishu chubanshe, 1988.

Dunhuang yiyao wenxian jijiao 敦煌醫藥文獻輯校. Edited by Ma Jixing 馬繼興 et al. Nanjing: Jiangsu guji chubanshe, 1998.

Ernian lüling yu zouyanshu: Zhangjiashan ersiqihao Han mu chutu falü wenxian shidu 二年律令與奏讞書: 張家山二四七號漢墓出土法律文獻釋讀. Edited by Peng Hao 彭浩, Chen Wei 陳偉, and Kudō Motoo 工藤元男. Shanghai: Shanghai guji, 2007.

Fan Ye 范曄 (398–445). *Hou Hanshu* 後漢書. Shanghai: Shanghai guji, 1986.

Fan Zhongyan 范仲淹 (989–1052). *Fan Zhongyan quanji* 范仲淹全集. Chengdu: Sichuan daxue chubanshe, 2002.

Fang Xuanling 房玄齡 (578–648) et al. *Jinshu* 晉書. Taipei: Dingwen shuju, 1980.

Fang Youzhi 方有執 (fl. 1589–99). *Shanghan lun tiaobian* 傷寒論條辨. Edited by Siku quanshu zhenben wuji 四庫全書珍本五集. Vols. 193–4. Taipei: Taiwan shangwu, 1974.

Feng Kebin 馮可賓 (fl. 1630) ed. *Guang Baichuan xuehai: fu suoyin* 廣百川學海: 附索引. Taipei: Xinxing shuju, 1970.

Gao Cheng 高承. *Shiwu jiyuan* 事物紀原. Edited by Congshu jicheng chubian 叢書集成初編. Vols. 1209–12. Shanghai: Shangwu yinshuguan, 1937.

Ge Hong 葛洪 (284–364). *Shenxian zhuan jiaoshi* 神仙傳校釋. Annotated by Hu Shouwei 胡守爲. Beijing: Zhonghua shuju, 2010.

Zhouhou beiji fang 肘後備急方. Changsha: Yuelu shushe, 1994.

Baopuzi neipian jiaoshi 抱朴子内篇校釋. Edited by Wang Ming 王明. Taipei: Liren shuju, 1981.

Guanju Qin Han mu jiandu 關沮秦漢墓簡牘. Beijing: Zhonghua shuju, 2001.

Gujin yishi. See Wang Honghan.

Gujin yitong daquan 古今醫統大全. Edited by Xu Chunfu 徐春甫 (1520–96). Renmin weisheng, 1991.

Guo Yong 郭雍 (1103–1187). *Zhongjing shanghan bu wang lun* 仲景傷寒補亡論. Ed Xuxiu siku quanshu 續修四庫全書. Vol. 984. Shanghai: Shanghai guji, 1995.

Guoyu 國語. Edited by Sibu beiyao 四部備要. Part 83. Shanghai: Zhonghua shuju, 1927–36.

Hanfei zi jijie 韓非子集解. Edited by Wang Xianshen 王先慎. Beijing: Zhonghua shuju, 1998.

Hanshu. See Ban Gu.

Heguazi 鶡冠子. Edited by Sibu beiyao 四部備要. Part 143. Annotated by Lu Dian 陸佃 (1042–1102). Shanghai: Zhonghua shuju, 1927–36.

Heguanzi huijiao jizhu: fu tong jian 鶡冠子彙校集注: 附通檢. Ed Huang Huaixin 黃懷信. Beijing: Zhonghua shuju, 2004.

Hou Hanshu. See Fan Ye.

Huainanzi 淮南子. Edited by Liu Wendian 劉文典. Beijing: Zhonghua, 1989.

Huangdi suwen lingshu jing 黃帝素問靈樞經. Edited by Sibu congkan 四部叢刊. Part 33. Shanghai: Shangwu yinshuguan, 1937–8.

Huangdi zhenjiu jiayi jing. See Huangfu Mi.

Huangfu Mi 皇甫謐 (215–82). *Zhenjiu jiayijing jiaozhu* 鍼灸甲乙經校注. 2 vols. Beijing: Renmin weisheng chubanshe, 1996.

Ishinpō. See Tanba Yasuyori.

Jiang Guan 江瓘 (1503–65). *Mingyi lei an* 名醫類案. Beijing: Renmin weisheng, 1957.

Jiayi jing. See Huangfu Mi.

Jinkui yaolüe. See Zhang Ji.

Jinshu. See Fang Xuanling et al.

Jiu Tangshu. See Liu Xu.

Juyan Hanjian shiwen hejiao 居延漢簡釋文合校. Edited by Xie Guihua 謝桂華 and Li Junming 李均明. 2 vols. Beijing: Wenwu, 1987.

Juyan xinjian: Jiaqu Houguan yu disi sui 居延新簡: 甲渠候官與第四燧. Beijing: Wenwu chubanshe, 1990.

Kangzhi ben Shanghan lun. See Zhang Ji.

Liang Yusheng 梁玉繩 (1744–1819). *Shiji zhiyi: fu lu* 史記志疑:附錄. 2 vols. Shanghai: Shangwu yinshuguan, 1937.

Lidai mingyi mengqiu. See Zhou Shouzhong.

Lienü zhuan. See Liu Xiang.

Li Fang 李昉 (925–96) et al. *Taiping yulan* 太平御覽. Taipei: Taiwan shangwu, 1975.

Taiping guangji 太平廣記. Beijing: Zhonghua, 1961. Rpt 1995.

Liji jijie 禮記集解. Annotated by Sun Xidan 孫希旦 (1736–84). Beijing: Zhonghua shuju, 1989. Rpt. 1998.

Li Lian 李濂 (1488–1566). *Yi shi* 醫史. Edited by Xuxiu siku quanshu 續修四庫全書. Vol. 1030. Shanghai: Shanghai guji, 2002.

Lingshu jing. See *Huangdi suwen lingshu jing*.

Liu Wansu 劉完素 (fl. 1186). *Suwen xuanji yuanbing shi* 素問玄機原病式. Edited by Sun Tong 孫桐. Nanjing: Jiangsu kexue jishu, 1985.

Liu Xiang 劉向 (77–6 BC). *Shuoyuan jinzhu jinyi* 說苑今註今譯. Comp. Lu Yuanjun 盧元駿. Taipei: Shangwu yinshuguan, 1988. Rpt. 1995.

Lienü zhuan jiaozhu 列女傳校注. Comp. Liang Duan 梁端. Edited by Sibu beiyao 四部備要. Part 93. Shanghai: Zhonghua shuju, 1927–36.

Liu Xiang 劉向 (77–6 BC) and Liu Xin 劉歆 (ca 46 BC–AD 23). *Qilüe bielu yiwen, qilüe yiwen* 七略別錄佚文. 七略佚文. Edited by Deng Junjie 鄧駿捷. Shanghai: Shanghai guji, 2008.

Liu Xu 劉昫 (887–946). *Jiu Tangshu* 舊唐書. Taipei: Dingwen shuju, 1981.

Liye Qin jian 里耶秦簡. Beijing: Wenwu chubanshe, 2012.

Liye Qin jiandu jiaoshi 里耶秦簡牘校釋. Edited by Chen Wei 陳偉, He Youzu 何有祖, Lu Jialiang 魯家亮, and Fan Guodong 凡國棟. Wuchang: Wuhan daxue chubanshe, 2012.

Lunheng. See Wang Chong.

Lunyu zhengyi 論語正義. Edited by Liu Baonan 劉寶楠 (1791–1855). 2 vols. Beijing: Zhonghua shuju, 1990. Rpt. 1998.

Lüshi chunqiu jiaoshi 吕氏春秋校釋. Edited by Chen Qiyou 陳奇猷. 2 vols. Shanghai: Xinhua shudian, 1983. Rpt. 1995.

Ma Duanlin 馬端臨 (ca. 1254–1323). *Wenxian tongkao* 文獻通考. Taipei: Taiwan shangwu yinshuguan, 1987.

Mawangdui gu yishu kaoshi 馬王堆古醫書考釋. Annotated by Ma Jixing 馬繼興. Changsha: Hunan kexue jishu chubanshe, 1992.

Mawangdui Han mu boshu 馬王堆漢墓帛書. Beijing: Wenwu chubanshe, 1985.

Mozi jiangu 墨子閒詁. Edited by Sun Yirang 孫詒讓 (1848–1908). Taipei: Huazheng shuju, 1987.

Nanjing benyi xinjie 難經本義新解. Edited by Lin Huizhen 林輝鎮. Taipei: Yiqun, 1986.

Ouyang Xiu 歐陽修 (1007–72) and Song Qi 宋祈 (998–1061). *Xin Tangshu* 新唐書. Taipei: Dingwen shuju, 1981.

Sanguo zhi. See Chen Shou.

Shanghai bowuguan cang Zhanguo Chu zhushu 上海博物館藏戰國楚竹書. Edited by Ma Chengyuan 馬承源. Shanghai: Shanghai guji, 2001–2008.

Shanghan lun banben daquan. See Zhang Ji.

Shanghan lun jiyi, Shanghan lunshu yi, Jinkui yuhan yaolüe jiyi, Jinkui yuhan yaolüe shuyi. See Zhang Ji.

Shenxian zhuan. See Ge Hong.

Shiji. See Sima Qian.

Shisan jing zhushu: fu jiaokan ji 十三經注疏: 附校勘記. Edited by Ruan Yuan 阮元 (1764–1849). Beijing: Zhonghua, 1980.

Shizi 尸子. Annotated by Wang Jipei 汪繼培 (b. 1775) and Sun Xingyan 孫星衍 (1753–1818). Edited by *Congshu jicheng* 叢書集成. Beijing: Zhonghua shuju, 1991.

Shuihudi Qin mu zhujian 睡虎地秦墓竹簡. Beijing: Wenwu chuban, 1990.

Shulehe liuyu chutu Hanjian 疏勒河流域出土漢簡. Edited by Lin Meicun 林梅村 and Li Junming 李均明. Beijing: Wenwu, 1984.

Shuowen. See Xu Shen.

Shuoyuan. See Liu Xiang.

Siku quanshu zongmu tiyao. See Yong Rong.

Sima Guang 司馬光 (1019–86). *Sima Guangji* 司馬光集. Edited by Li Wenze 李文澤 and Xia Shaohui 霞紹暉. 3 vols. Chengdu: Sichuan daxue, 2010.

Sima Qian 司馬遷 (145–ca. 86 BC). *Shiji* 史記. Annotated by Pei Yin 裴駰 (fl. 438). Taipei: Dingwen shuju, 1981.

Songshi. See Tuotuo.

Suishu. See Wei Zheng.

Sun Simiao 孙思邈 (581–682). *Sun Zhenren qianjin fang: fu zhenben qianjin fang* 孫真人千金方: 附真本千金方. Beijing: Renmin weisheng. 1996.

Beiji qianjin yaofang 備急千金要方. Taipei: Zhongguo yiyao yanjiusuo, 1990.

Qianjin yifang 千金翼方. Taipei: Zhongguo yiyao yanjiusuo, 1974.

Taiping guangji. See Li Fang et al.

Taiping yulan. See Li Fang et al.

Takigawa Kametarō 瀧川龜太郎 (b. 1865). *Shiki kaichū kōshō fu kōho* 史記會注考證附校補. 2 vols. Shanghai: Shanghai guji, 1986.

Taki Mototane 多紀元胤 (1789–1827). *Zhongguo yijikao* 中國醫籍考. Beijing: Renmin weisheng, 1956.

Tanba Yasuyori 丹波康頼 (912–95). *Ishinpō* 醫心方. Shenyang: Liaoning kexue jishu, 1996.

Ishinpō 醫心方. Annotated and translated into Japanese by Maki Sachiko 槇佐知子. 33 vols. Tokyo: Chikuma Shobō, 1993–2012.

Tongzhi. See Zheng Qiao.

Tuotuo 脫脫 (1313–1355). *Songshi* 宋史. Taipei: Dingwen shuju, 1980.

Waitai miyao. See Wang Tao.

Wang Chong 王充 (ca. 27–97). *Lunheng jiaoshi* 論衡校釋. Edited by Huang Hui 黃暉. Beijing: Zhonghua shuju, 1990.

Wang Honghan 王宏翰 (17th cent.). *Gujin yishi* 古今醫史. Edited by Xuxiu Siku quanshu 續修四庫全書. Vol. 1030. Shanghai: Shanghai guji, 2002.

Wang Qinruo 王欽若 (962–1025) et al. *Cefu yuangui* 冊府元龜. Beijing: Zhonghua shuju, 1984.

Wang Tao 王燾 (8th cent.). *Waitai miyao* 外臺秘要. Taipei: Zhongguo yiyao yanjiusuo, 1965.

Wei Zheng 魏徵 (580–643) et al. *Suishu* 隋書. Beijing: Zhonghua shuju, 1973. Rpt. 2000.

Wu Cheng 吳澄 (1249–1333). *Wu Wenzheng ji* 吳文正集. Edited by Siku quanshu zhenben erji 四庫全書珍本二集. Vols. 319–28. Taipei: Taiwan shangwu yinshuguan, 1971.

Wuwei Handai yi jian 武威漢代醫簡. Edited by Gansusheng bowuguan 甘肅省博物館. Beijing: Zhonghua shuju, 1975.

Wuwei Handai yi jian zhujie 武威漢代醫簡注解. Edited by Zhang Yanchang 張延昌. Beijing: Zhongyi guji chubanshe, 2006.

Xin Tangshu. See Ouyang Xiu and Song Qi.

Xinji Songben shanghan lun. See Zhang Ji.

Xu Shen 許慎 (fl. ca. 121). *Shuowen jiezi zhu* 說文解字注. Shanghai: Shanghai guji, 1981.

Xu Shuwei 許叔微 (fl. 1132). *Leizheng puji benshi fang* 類證普濟本事方. Edited by Siku quanshu zhenben wuji 四庫全書珍本五集. Vols. 166–7. Taipei: Taiwan shangwu yinshuguan, 1974.

Yang Jizhou 楊繼洲 (1573–1619). *Zhenjiu dacheng* 針灸大成. Edited by Xuxiu Siku quanshu 續修四庫全書. Vol. 996. Shanghai: Shanghai guji chubanshe, 2002.

Yanzi chunqiu 晏子春秋. Edited by Sibu bei yao 四部備要. Pt. 90. Shanghai: Zhonghua shuju, 1927–36.

Yibu quanlu 醫部全錄. Edited by Chen Menglei 陳夢雷 (1650–1741) et al. Beijing: Renmin weisheng, 1998.

Yinwan Hanmu jiandu jiaoli 尹灣漢墓簡牘校理. Edited by Zhang Xiancheng 張顯成 and Zhou Qunli 周群麗. Tianjin: Tianjin guji chubanshe, 2011.

Yi shi. See Li Lian.

Yi shuo. See Zhang Gao and Yu Bian.

Yong Rong 永瑢 (1744–1790) et al. *Siku quanshu zongmu tiyao* 四庫全書總目提要. Shanghai: Shangwu yinshuguan, 1933.

Yu Chang 喻昌 (17th cent.). *Shanglun pian* 尚論篇. Edited by Siku quanshu zhenben erji 四庫全書珍本二集. Vols. 192–3. Taipei: Taiwan shangwu yinshuan, 1971.

Yuelu shuyuan cang Qin jian 嶽麓書院藏秦簡. Vol. 3. Edited by Zhu Hanmin 朱漢民 and Chen Songchang 陳松長. Shanghai: Shanghai cishu chubanshe, 2013.

Zhanguo ce 戰國策. Edited by Sibu beiyao 四部備要. Part 84. Shanghai: Zhonghua shuju, 1927–36.

Zhanguo ce zhushi 戰國策注釋. Edited by He Jianzhang 何建章. Beijing: Zhonghua shuju, 1990. Rpt. 1991.

Zhang Gao 張杲 (12th–13th cent.) and Yu Bian 俞弁 (16th cent.). *Yi shuo* 醫說. Edited by Siku quanshu zhenben liuji 四庫全書珍本六集. Vols. 193–4. Taipei: Taiwan shangwu yinshuguan, 1976.

Zhang Ji 張機 or Zhang Zhongjing 張仲景 (2nd–3rd cent. AD). *Zhongjing quanshu* 仲景全書. Edited by Zhao Kaimei 趙開美 (fl. ca. 1599). Beijing: Guyi guji chubanshe, 2004.

Jinkui yaolüe 金匱要略. Edited by Li Keguang 李克光. Taipei: Zhiyin, 2002.

Shanghanlun banben daquan 傷寒論版本大全. Edited by Li Shunbao 李順保. Beijing: Xueyuan chubanshe, 2001.

Shanghan lun jiyi, Shanghan lunshu yi, Jinkui yuhan yaolüe jiyi, Jinkui yuhan yaolüe shuyi 傷寒論輯義. 傷寒論述義. 金匱玉函要略輯義. 金匱玉函要略述義. Edited by Tamba Motoyasu 丹波元簡 (1755–1810). Beijing: Renmin weisheng, 1983.

Kangzhi ben Shanghan lun 康治本傷寒論. Edited by Togami Genhi 戶上玄斐. Beijing: Zhongyi guji, 1982.

Zhujie Shanghan lun 注解傷寒論. Edited by Cheng Wuji 成無己 (1063–1156). Taipei: Yiwen, 1967.

Xinji Songben shanghan lun 新輯宋本傷寒論. Chongqing: Chongqing renmin chuban, 1955.

Zhangjiashan Han mu zhujian 張家山漢墓竹簡. Beijing: Wenwu chubanshe, 2001. Rpt. 2006.

Zheng Qiao 鄭樵 (1104–62). *Tongzhi* 通志. Taipei: Taiwan shangwu yinshuguan, 1987.

Zhenjiu jiayi jing. See Huangfu Mi.

Zhongguo yiji kao. See Taki Mototane.

Zhongjing quanshu. See Zhang Ji.

Zhou Shouzhong 周守忠 (fl. 1208). *Lidai mingyi mengqiu* 歷代名醫蒙求. Edited by Xuxiu Siku quanshu 續修四庫全書. Vol. 1030. Shanghai: Shanghai guji, 2002.

Zuozhuan zhushu 左傳注疏. Edited by Sibu beiyao 四部備要. Part 20. Vols. 137–56. Shanghai: Zhonghua shuju, 1927–36.

Zhubing yuanhou lun. See Chao Yuanfang.

Zhujie Shanghan lun. See Zhang Ji.

Zhu Danxi 朱丹溪 (1281–1358). *Danxi xinfa* 丹溪心法. Shenyang: Liaoning kexue jishu, 1997.

REFERENCES POST-1900

Andrews, Bridie. 2014. *The Making of Modern Chinese Medicine, 1850–1960*. Vancouver: University of British Columbia Press.

2013. "The Republic of China." In *Chinese Medicine and Healing: An Illustrated History*, edited by T. J. Hinrichs and Linda L. Barnes, 209–38. Cambridge, MA: Belknap Press of Harvard University Press.

1997. "Tuberculosis and the Assimilation of Germ Theory in China, 1895–1937." *Journal of the History of Medicine and the Allied Sciences* 52.1: 114–57.

Biagioli, Mario. 2006. *Galileo's Instruments of Credit: Telescopes, Images, Secrecy*. Chicago: Chicago University Press.

Blackburn, Anne M. 2001. *Buddhist Learning and Textual Practice in Eighteenth-Century Sri Lankan Monastic Culture*. Princeton, NJ: Princeton University Press.

Boyanton, Stephen. Forthcoming. "The *Treatise on Cold Damage* and the Formation of Literati Medicine: Social, Epidemiological, and Medical Change in China, 1000–1400." PhD diss., Columbia University.

Bridgman, R. F. 1955. "La médecine dans la Chine antique." *Mélanges Chinois et Bouddhiques* 10: 1–213.

Brown, Miranda. 2013. "Mozi's Remaking of Ancient Authority." In *The Mozi as an Evolving Text: Different Voices in Early Chinese Thought*, edited by Carine Defoort and Nicolas Standaert, 143–74. Leiden, The Netherlands: Brill.

2012. "Who Was He? Reflections on China's First Medical 'Naturalist.'" *Medical History* 56.3: 366–89.

2006. "Neither 'Primitive' nor 'Others,' But Somehow Not Quite Like 'Us': The Fortunes of Psychic Unity and Essentialism in Chinese Studies." *Journal of the Economic and Social History of the Orient* 49.2: 219–52.

Brown, Miranda, and Uffe Bergeton. 2008. "'Seeing' Like a Sage: Three Takes on Identity and Perception." *Journal of Chinese Philosophy* 35.4: 641–62.

Brown, Miranda, and Charles Sanft. 2011. "Categories and Legal Reasoning in Early Imperial China: The Meaning of *Fa* in Recovered Texts." *Oriens Extremus* 49: 283–306.

Cai, Liang. 2011. "Excavating the Genealogy of Classical Studies in the Western Han Dynasty (206 BCE–8 CE)." *Journal of the American Oriental Society* 131.1: 371–94.

Campany, Robert Ford. 2009. *Making Transcendants: Ascetics and Social Memory in Early Medieval China*. Honolulu: University of Hawaii Press.

Chaffee, John. 1995. *The Thorny Gates of Learning in Sung China: A Social History of Examinations*. Albany: State University of New York Press.

Chao, Yuan-ling. 2009. *Medicine and Society in Late Imperial China: A Study of Physicians in Suzhou, 1600–1850*. New York: Peter Lang.

Chen Bangxian 陳邦賢. 1937. *Zhongguo yixue shi* 中國醫學史. Shanghai: Shangwu yinshuguan.

Chen Bangxian 陳邦賢, and Yan Lingzhou 嚴菱舟. 1956. *Zhongguo yixue renming zhi* 中國醫學人名誌. Beijing: Renmin weisheng.

Chen Cunren 陳存仁. 1968. *Zhongguo yixueshi* 中國醫學史. Hong Kong: Chinese Medical Institute.

Chen Ning. 2000. "The Etymology of *Sheng* (Sage) and Its Confucian Conception in Early China." *Journal of Chinese Philosophy* 27.4: 409–27.

Chen Senhe 陳森和, and Ouyang Yu'e 歐陽玉娥. 2010. "Zhongjing xuwen yingxi houren tuozuo yu Sun Simiao zhi hou, Wang Bing zhi qian" 仲景序文應係後人託作於孫思邈之後,王冰之前. *Zhongyiyao yanjiu luncong* 中醫藥研究論叢 13.1: 25–42.

Chen Songchang 陳松長. 2009. "Yuelu shuyuan suocang Qin jin zongshu" 岳麓書院所藏秦簡綜述. *Wenwu* 文物 2009.3: 75–88.

Chen Wei 陳偉. 2007. "'Jian dawang bo han'" xinyan 《簡大王泊旱》新研. *Jianbo* 簡帛 2: 259–68.

Chen Yuan 陳垣. 1958. *Shihui juli* 史諱舉例. Beijing: Kexueyuan chubanshe.

Chen Yuanpeng 陳元朋. 1997. *Liang Song de "shang yi shiren" yu "ruyi": jianlun qi zai Jin Yuan de liubian* 兩宋的「尚醫士人」與「儒醫」: 兼論其在金元的流變. Taipei: Guoli Taiwan daxue.

Chen Zhi 陳直. 1988. *Wenshi kaogu luncong* 文史考古論叢. Tianjin: Tianjin guji.

Cherniack, Susan. 1994. "Book Culture and Textual Transmission in Sung China." *Harvard Journal of Asiatic Studies* 54.1: 5–125.

Clunas, Craig. 1997. Rpt. 2009. *Art in China*, 2nd Edition. Oxford and New York: Oxford University Press.

Cook, Constance. 2013. "The Dreams of the Lord of Jin." In *Chinese Medicine and Healing: An Illustrated History*, edited by T. J. Hinrichs and Linda L Barnes, 18–20. Cambridge, MA: Belknap Press of Harvard University Press.

2006. *Death in Ancient China: The Tale of One Man's Journey*. Leiden, The Netherlands: Brill.

Croizier, Ralph C. 1968. *Traditional Medicine in Modern China: Science, Nationalism, and the Tensions of Cultural Change*. Cambridge, MA: Harvard University Press.

Csikszentmihalyi, Mark. 2002. "Traditional Taxonomies and Revealed Texts in the Han." In *Daoist Identity: History, Lineage, and Ritual*, edited by Livia Kohn and Harold Roth, 81–101. Honolulu: University of Hawai'i Press.

2004. *Material Virtue: Ethics and the Body in Early China*. Leiden, The Netherlands: Brill.

2006. *Readings in Han Chinese Thought*. Indianapolis: Hackett.

Csikszentmihalyi, Mark, and Michael Nylan. 2003. "Constructing Lineages and Inventing Traditions through Exemplary Figures in Early China." *T'oung Pao* 89: 59–99.

Cullen, Christopher. 2001. "*Yi'an* (case statements): the Origins of a Genre of Chinese Medical Literature." In *Innovation in Chinese Medicine*, edited by Elisabeth Hsu, 297–323. Cambridge: Cambridge University Press.

DeClercq, Dominik. 1998. *Writing Against the State: Political Rhetorics in Third and Fourth Century China*. Leiden, The Netherlands: Brill.

DeCrespigny, Rafe. 2007. *Biographical Dictionary of Later Han to the Three Kingdoms (23–220 AD)*. Leiden, The Netherlands: Brill.

2010. *Imperial Warlord: A Biography of Cao Cao 155–220 AD*. Leiden, The Netherlands: Brill.

Defoort, Carine. 2001a. "Is There Such a Thing as Chinese Philosophy? Arguments of an Implicit Debate." *Philosophy East and West* 51.3: 393–413.

2001b. "Ruling the World with Words: The Idea of *Zhengming* in the *Shizi*." *Bulletin of the Museum of Far Eastern Antiquities* 7:3: 217–42.

1997. *The Pheasant Cap Master: He guan zi, A Rhetorical Reading*. Albany: State University of New York Press.

Denecke, Wiebke. 2010. *The Dynamics of the Masters Literature: Early Chinese Thought from Confucius to Han Feizi*. Cambridge, MA: Harvard University Asia Center.

DeWoskin, Kenneth J. 1983. *Doctors, Diviners, and Magicians of Ancient China: Biographies of Fang-shih*. New York: Columbia University Press.

Dirks, Nicholas B. 2001. *Castes of Mind: Colonialism and the Making of Modern India*. Princeton, NJ: Princeton University Press.

Dong Fayao 董法堯. 2012. "Huangdi neijing chengshu yanjiu" 黃帝內經成書研究. MA thesis, Shandong shifan daxue.

Dong Muda 董慕達 [Miranda Brown]. 2007. "Qinggan yu siwei de weizhi: Lun gudai wenxianzhong de 'ganqing'" 情感與思維的位置: 論古代文獻中的'肝情. *Yuandao* 道原 13 (2007): 237–48.

Duan Yishan 段逸山 et al. comp. 1986. Rpt. 1994. *Yi guwen* 醫古文. Beijing: Renmin weisheng chubanshe.

Durrant, Stephen W. 1995. *The Cloudy Mirror: Tension and Conflict in the Writings of Sima Qian.* Albany: State University of New York Press.

Du Zhengsheng 杜正勝. 1995. "Zuowei shehuishi de yiliaoshi – bing jieshao jibing, yiliao yu wenhua yantao xiaozu de chengguo" 作為社會史的醫療史 – 並介紹疾病, 醫療與文化研討小組的成果. *Xinshi xue* 新史學 6.1: 113–53.

Eaton, Richard M. 2000. "(Re)imag(in)ing Other²ness: A Postmortem for the Postmodern in India." *Journal of World History* 11.1 (2000): 57–78.

Ebrey, Patricia. 2010. *The Cambridge Illustrated History of China, 2nd ed.* Cambridge: Cambridge University Press.

Egan, Ronald. 1977. "Narratives in Tso Chuan." *Harvard Journal of Asiatic Studies* 37.2: 323–52.

Elstein, David. 2006. "Friend or Father? Competing Visions of Master-Student Relations in Early China." PhD diss., University of Michigan.

Epler, Deane C., Jr. 1977. "The Concept of Disease in Two Third Century Chinese Medical Texts." PhD diss., University of Washington.

Fan Jiawei 范家偉 [Fan Ka Wai]. 2013. "The Period of Division and the Tang Period." In *Chinese Medicine and Healing: An Illustrated History*, edited by T. J. Hinrichs and Linda L. Barnes, 65–96. Cambridge, MA: Belknap Press of Harvard University Press.

2010a. *Zhonggu shiqi de yizhe yu bingzhe* 中古时期的醫者與病者. Shanghai: Fudan daxue.

2010b. "Songdai yixue fazhan de waiyuan yinsu – ping Guo Zhisong Zhong yiyao de yanbian: Songdai (960–1200)" 宋代醫學發展的外緣因素–評郭志松 《中醫藥的演變: 宋代 (960–1200 年) 》. *Zhongguo kejishi zazhi* 中國科技史雜志 31.3 (2010): 328–36.

2007. *Da yi jingcheng: Tangdai guojia, xinyang yu yixue* 大醫精誠: 唐代國家、信仰與醫學. Taipei: Dongda tushu.

2004. *Liuchao Sui Tang yixue zhi chuancheng yu zhenghe* 六朝隋唐醫學之傳承與整合. Hong Kong: Chinese University Press.

Fan Ka wai [Fan Jiawei] and Sze-nga Lau. 2010. "Review of *The Evolution of Chinese Medicine*, Song Dynasty, 960–1200 by Asaf Goldschmidt." *The International Journal of Asian Studies* 7.2: 232–5.

Fan Xingzhun 范行準. 1986. *Zhongguo yixue shilüe* 中國醫學史略. Beijing: Zhongyi guji chubanshe.

Farquhar, Judith. 1994. *Knowing Practice: The Clinical Encounter of Chinese Medicine*. Boulder, CO: Westview Press.

Fischer, Paul. 2009. "Intertextuality in Early Chinese Master-Texts: Shared Narratives in *Shi Zi*." *Asia Major*, 3rd Series 22.2: 1–34.

Flohr, Carsten. 1996. "The Plague Fighter: Wu Lien-teh and the Beginning of the Chinese Public Health System." *Annals of Science* 53 (1996): 361–80.

Freidson, Eliot. 1970. *Profession of Medicine: A Study of the Sociology of Applied Knowledge*. New York: Dodd, Mead.

Furth, Charlotte. 2007. "Introduction: Thinking with Cases." In *Thinking with Cases: Specialist Knowledge in Chinese Cultural History*, edited by Charlotte Furth, Judith T. Zeitlin, and Hsiung Ping-chen, 1–27. Honolulu: University of Hawaii Press.

1999. *A Flourishing Yin: Gender in China's Medical History, 960–1665*. Berkeley: University of California Press.

Gansusheng bowuguan 甘肅省博物館, and Gansusheng Wuweixian wenhuaguan 甘肅省武威縣文化館. 1973. "Wuwei Hantanpo Hanmu fajue jianbao – chutu dapi yiyao jiandu" 武威旱灘坡漢墓發掘簡報 -- 出土大批醫藥簡牘. *Wenwu* 文物 1973.12: 18–22.

Giradot, Norman J. 2002. *The Victorian Translation of China: James Legge's Oriental Pilgrimage*. Berkeley: University of California Press.

Goldschmidt, Asaf. 2009. *The Evolution of Chinese Medicine, Song Dynasty, 960–1200*. London: Routledge.

Hallisey, Charles. 1995. "Roads Taken and Not Taken in the Study of Theravada Buddhism." In *Curators of the Buddha: The Study of Buddhism under Colonialism*, edited by Donald S. Lopez Jr., 31–61. Chicago: University of Chicago Press.

Han Jianping 韓健平. 2007. "Chuanshuo de shenyi: Bian Que" 傳說的神醫: 扁鵲. *Kexue wenhua pinglun* 科學文化評論 4.5: 5–14.

Hanson, Marta. 2011. *Speaking of Epidemics in Chinese Medicine: Disease and the Geographic Imagination in Late Imperial China*. London and New York: Routledge.

2003. "The *Golden Mirror* in the Imperial Court of the Qianlong Emperor, 1739–1742." *Early Science and Medicine* 8.2: 111–47.

Harper, Donald. 2010. "The Textual Form of Knowledge: Occult Miscellanies in Ancient and Medieval Chinese Manuscripts, Fourth Century BC to Tenth Century AD." In *Looking at It from Asia: The Processes That Shaped the Sources of History of Science*, edited by Florence Bretelle-Establet, 37–80. Dordrecht, The Netherlands: Springer.

2001. "Iatromancy, Diagnosis, and Prognosis in Early Chinese Medicine." In *Innovation in Chinese Medicine*, edited by Elisabeth Hsu, 99–120. Cambridge: Cambridge University Press.

1998. *Early Chinese Medical Literature: The Mawangdui Medical Manuscripts.* London and New York: Kegan Paul International.

Hart, Roger. 1999. "Beyond Science and Civilisation: a Post-Needham Critique." *East Asia Science, Technology, and Medicine* 16: 88–114.

Hinrichs, T. J. 2013. "A Late Han Adept." In *Chinese Medicine and Healing: An Illustrated History*, edited by T. J. Hinrichs and Linda L. Barnes, 53–5. Cambridge, MA: Belknap Press of Harvard University Press.

1998. "New Geographies of Chinese Medicine." *Osiris, 2nd Series, Beyond Joseph Needham: Science, Technology, and Medicine in East and Southeast Asia* 13: 287–325.

Ho Peng Yoke. 2007. *Explorations in Daoism: Medicine and Alchemy in Literature.* London: Routledge.

Hsia, R. Po-chia. 2010. *A Jesuit in a Forbidden City: Matteo Ricci, 1552–1610.* Oxford: Oxford University Press.

Hsiung, Ping-chen. 2007. "Facts in Tales: Case Records and Pediatric Medicine in Late Imperial China." In *Thinking with Cases: Specialist Knowledge in Chinese Cultural History*, edited by Charlotte Furth, Judith T. Zeitlin, and Hsiung Ping-chen, 152–68. Honolulu: University of Hawai'i Press.

Hsu, Elisabeth. 2010. *Pulse Diagnosis in Early China: The Telling Touch.* Cambridge: Cambridge University Press.

Hulsewé, A. F. P. 1985. *Remnants of Ch'in Law: An Annotated Translation of the Ch'in Legal and Administrative Rules of the 3rd Century B.C., Discovered in Yün-meng Prefecture, Hu-pei Province, in 1975.* Leiden, The Netherlands: Brill.

1975. "The Problem of the Authenticity of 'Shih-chi' Chapter 123, the Memoir of Ta Yüan." *T'oung Pao* 61: 83–147.

Hu Shui-ying. 1999. *An Enumeration of Chinese Materia Medica*, 2nd Edition. Hong Kong: Chinese University of Hong Kong Press.

Hymes, Robert. 1987. "Not Quite Gentlemen: Doctors in the Sung and Yuan." *Chinese Science* 8: 9–76.

1986. *Statesmen and Gentlemen: The Elite of Fu-chou, Chiang-hsi, in Northern and Southern Song.* Cambridge: Cambridge University Press.

Jensen, Lionel. 1997. *Manufacturing Confucianism: Chinese Traditions and Universal Civilization.* Durham, NC: Duke University Press.

Jiang Dianwei 姜殿偉. 2003. "Yi He shi gu – du 'Qin Yi Huan He' zhaji" 醫和釋蠱–讀《秦醫緩和》札記. *Liaoning zhongyi xueyuan xuebao* 遼寧中醫學院學報 5.4: 414.

Jin Shiqi 金仕起. 2005. "Gudai yizhe de juese – jian lun qi shenfen yu diwei" 古代醫者的角色-兼論其身份與地位. In *Shengming yu yiliao* 生命與醫療, edited by Li Jianmin 李建民, 1–35. Beijing: Zhongguo dabaike quanshu chubanshe.

2009. "Jin Pinggong bing an gouchen 晉平公病案鉤沉." *Guoli zhengzhi daxue lishi xuebao* 國立政治大學歷史學報 31.5: 1–50.

2010. *Zhongguo gudai de yixue, yishi yu zhengzhi: yi yishi wenben wei zhongxin de yi ge fenxi* 中國古代的醫學、醫史與政治：以醫史文本為中心的一個分析. Taipei: Zhengda chubanshe.

Kalinowski, Marc. 2010. "Divination and Astrology: Received Texts and Excavated Manuscripts." In *China's Early Empires: A Re-Appraisal*, edited by Michael Nylan and Michael Loewe, 339–66. Cambridge: Cambridge University Press.

2009. "Diviners and Astrologers under the Eastern Zhou: Transmitted Texts and Recent Archaeological Discoveries." In *Early Chinese Religion, Part One: Shang through Han (1250 BC–220 AD)*, edited by John Lagerwey and Marc Kalinowski, I: 341–96. Leiden, The Netherlands, and Boston: Brill.

1999. "La rhétorique oraculaire dans les chroniques anciennes de la China: Une étude des discours prédictifs dans le Zuozhuan." In *Divination et rationalité en Chine ancienne. Extrême-Orient, Extrême-Occident*, edited by Karine Chemla, Donald Harper, and Marc Kalinowski, 21. 37–65. Paris: Centre national du livre.

Keegan, David. 1988. "The 'Huang-ti Nei-ching': The Structure of the Compilation: The Significance of the Structure." PhD diss., University of California, Berkeley.

Knapp, Keith N. 2000. "Heaven and Death According to Huangfu Mi, A Third-Century Confucian." *Early Medieval China* 6: 1–31.

Knechtges, David R. 1993. "*Ho-kuan-tzu*." In *Early Chinese Texts: A Bibliographical Guide*, edited by Michael Loewe, 137–40. Berkeley: Society for the Study of Early China.

Klein, Esther. 2010. "History of a Historian: Perspectives on the Authorial Roles of Sima Qian." PhD diss., Princeton University.

Kuhn, Dieter, and Timothy Brook. 2009. *The Age of Confucian Rule: The Song Transformation of China*. Cambridge, MA: Belknap.

Kuriyama Shigehisa. 1999. Rpt. 2002. *The Expressiveness of the Body and the Divergence of Greek and Chinese Medicine*. New York: Zone Books.

Lai Guolong 來國龍. 2011a. "'Jian dawang bohan' de xushi jiegou yu zongjiao beijing – jianshi 'shaji'" 《柬大王泊旱》的敘事結構與宗教背景–兼釋"殺祭". *Proceedings for the Second International Forum on Excavated Manuscripts at the National Taiwan University, Taipei, Taiwan*. 433–74. Taipei: Taiwan daxue chubanshe.

2011b. "Lun Chu bushi jidao jian zhong de 'yudao'" 論楚卜筮祭禱簡中的"與禱. *Jianbo* 簡帛 6: 359–78.

2005. "Death and the Otherworldly Journey in Early China as Seen through Tomb Texts, Travel Paraphernalia, and Road Rituals." *Asia Major*, 3rd Series 18.1: 1–44.

Lee T'ao [Li Tao]. 1953. "Achievements of Chinese Medicine in the Ch'in (221–207 B.C.) and Han (206 B.C.–219 A.D.) Dynasties." *Chinese Medical Journal* 71: 380–96.

1940. "Ten Celebrated Physicians and their Temples." *Chinese Medical Journal* 58: 267–74.

Lei, Sean Hsiang-lin. 2009. "Moral Community of *Weisheng*: Contesting Hygiene in Republican China." *East Asian Science, Technology and Society: An International Journal* 3:475–504.

2002. "How Did Chinese Medicine Become Experiential? The Political Epistemology of *Jingyan*." *Positions: East Asian Cultures Critique* 10.2: 333–64.

Forthcoming. "Living Tradition and Local Innovation: Making Meaning and Articulating Reality in Asian STS." Paper Presented at the International Workshop on "Toward a Trans-Asian Science and Technology Studies," Asian Research Institute and Science, Technology and Society Cluster, National University of Singapore, March 6, 2009.

Leung, Angela Li-Che. 2013. "The Yuan and Ming Periods." In *Chinese Medicine and Healing: An Illustrated History*, edited by T. J. Hinrichs and Linda L. Barnes, 129–59. Cambridge, MA: Belknap Press of Harvard University Press.

2003. "Medical Learning from the Song to Ming." In *The Song-Yuan-Ming Transition in Chinese History*, edited by Paul Jackov Smith and Richard von Glahn, 374–98. Cambridge, MA: Harvard University Asia Center.

Levi, Jean. 1999. "Pratiques divinatoires, conjectures et critiques rationalistes à l'époque des Royaumes Combattants." *Extrême-Orient, Extrême-Occident* 21: 67–77. Paris: Centre national du livre.

Lévi-Strauss, Claude. 1966. *Savage Mind*. Chicago: University of Chicago Press.

1962. Rpt. 1991. *Totemism*. Trans. Rodney Needham. London: Merlin Press.

Lewis, Mark Edward. 1999. "Warring States Political History." In *Cambridge History of Ancient China: From the Origins of Civilization to 221 BC*, edited by Michael Loewe and Edward Shaughnessy, 587–650. Cambridge: Cambridge University Press.

Liao Boyuan 廖伯源. 2008. *Qin Han shi luncong* 秦漢史論叢. Beijing: Zhonghua shuju.

Liao Yuqun 廖育群. 2011. *Traditional Chinese Medicine*. Trans. Li Zhaoguo et al. Cambridge: Cambridge University Press.

1996. *Zhongguo gudai kexue jishu shigang. Yixue juan* 中國古代科學技术史綱. 醫學卷. Shenyang: Liaoning jiaoyu chubanshe.

Li Bocong 李伯聰. 1990. *Bian Que he Bian Que xuepai yanjiu* 扁鵲和扁鵲學派研究. Xi'an: Shaanxi kexue jishu chubanshe.

Li Hongfu 李洪甫. 1982. "Jiangsu Lianyungang shi Huaguoshan chutu de Handai jiandu" 江蘇連雲港市花果山出土的漢代簡牘. *Kaogu* 考古 1982.5: 476–80.

Li Jianmin 李建民. 2000. *Sisheng zhi yu: Zhou Qin Han maixue zhi yuanliu* 死生之域: 周秦漢脈學之源流. Taipei: Zhongyang yanjiuyuan lishi yuyan yanjiusuo.

Li Jingwei 李經緯. 2007. *Zhongyi shi* 中醫史. Yihaikou: Hainan chubanshe.

Li Junming 李均明. 2009. *Qin Han jiandu wenshu fenlei jijie* 秦漢簡牘文書分類輯解. Beijing: Wenwu.

Li Ling 李零. 2000. *Zhongguo fangshu kao* 中國方術考. Beijing: Dongfang chubanshe.

Liu Boji 劉伯驥. 1974. *Zhongguo yixueshi* 中國醫學史.Yangming shan: Huagang chubanshe.

Liu Hainian 劉海年 and Yang Yifan 楊一凡. 1994. *Zhongguo zhenxi falü dianji jicheng* 中國珍稀法律典籍集成. 5 vols. Beijing: Kexue chubanshe.

Liu Lexian 劉樂賢. 2007. "Liye Qin jian he Kongjiapo Hanjian zhong de zhiguan shengcheng" 里耶秦簡和孔家坡漢簡中的職官省稱. *Wenwu* 文物 2007.9: 93–6.

Liu, Lydia. 1995. *Translingual Practice: Literature, National Culture, Translated Modernity, China, 1900–1937.* Stanford, CA: Stanford University Press.

Liu Renyuan 劉仁遠, Han Lijun 韓立軍, and Wu Chenggui 吳承貴. 2002. *Bian Que huikao* 扁鵲彙考. Beijing: Junshi yixue kexue.

Liu Xinfang 劉信芳. 2011. *Chuxi jianbo shili* 楚系簡帛釋例. Hefei: Anhui daxue chubanshe.

Liu Zhiqing 劉芝慶. 2009. "Xiushen yu zhiguo: cong Xianqin zhuzi dao Xihan qianqi shenti zhengzhi lun de shanbian" 修身與治國:從先秦諸子到西漢前期身體政治論的嬗變. MA thesis, History Dept. Taiwan daxue.

Li Wai-yee. 2007. *The Readability of the Past in Early Chinese Historiography.* Cambridge, MA: Harvard University Asia Center.

Lloyd, Geoffrey. 2010. "The Techniques of Persuasion and the Rhetoric of Disorder in Late Zhanguo and Western Han Texts." In *China's Early Empires: A Reappraisal*, edited by Michael Nylan and Michael Loewe, 451–60. Cambridge: Cambridge University Press.

2004. *In the Grip of Disease: Studies in the Greek Imagination.* Oxford: Oxford University Press.

1996. *Authorities and Adversaries: Investigations into Ancient Greek and Chinese Science.* Cambridge: Cambridge University Press.

Lloyd, Geoffrey, and Nathan Sivin. 2002. *The Way and the Word: Science and Medicine in Early China and Greece.* New Haven, CT: Yale University Press.

Lo, Vivienne. 2014. *How to Do the Gibbon Walk: A Translation of the Pulling Book (ca. 186 BCE).* Cambridge: Needham Research Institute Working Papers.

2013. "The Han Period." In *Chinese Medicine and Healing: An Illustrated History*, edited by T. J. Hinrichs and Linda L. Barnes, 31–64. Cambridge, MA: Belknap Press of Harvard University Press.

1998. "The Influence of *Yangsheng* Culture on Early Chinese Medical Theory." PhD diss., School of Oriental and African Studies.

Lo, Vivienne, and Christopher Cullen eds. 2005. *Medieval Chinese Medicine: The Dunhuang Medical Manuscripts.* London: Routledge.

Lo, Vivienne, and Li Jianmin. 2010. "Manuscripts, Received Texts, and the Healing Arts." In *China's Early Empires: A Reappraisal*, edited by Michael Nylan and Michael Loewe, 367–97. Cambridge: Cambridge University Press.

Loewe, Michael. 2014. "Liu Xiang and Liu Xin." *Chang'an 26 BCE: An Augustan Age in China*, edited by Griet VanKeerberghen and Michael Nylan. Seattle: University of Washington Press.

2011. *Bing: From Farmer's Son to Magistrate in Han China*. Indianapolis: Hackett Publishing.

1997. "The Physician Chunyu Yi and his Historical Background." In *En suivant la voie royale: mélanges offerts en hommage à Léon Vendermeersch*. Études Thématiques 7, edited by Jacques Gernet and Marc Kalinowski, 297–313. Paris: École Française d'Extrême-Orient.

Loewe, Michael, and Edward L. Shaughnessy, eds. 1999. *The Cambridge History of Ancient China: From the Origins of Civilization to 221 B.C.* Cambridge: Cambridge University Press.

Low, Morris E. 1998. "Introduction." *Osiris, 2nd Series, Beyond Joseph Needham: Science, Technology, and Medicine in East and Southeast Asia* 13: 1–8.

Lu Gwei-djen, and Joseph Needham. 1980. *Celestial Lancets: A History and Rationale of Acupuncture and Moxa*. Cambridge: Cambridge University Press.

Lu Xun 魯迅. 1960. *Selected Stories of Lu Hsun*. Translated by Yang Hsien-Yi and Gladys Yang. Beijing: Foreign Languages Press.

Ma Boying 馬伯英. 1994. *Zhongguo yixue wenhua shi* 中國醫學文化史. Shanghai renmin chubanshe.

Ma Jixing 馬繼興. 2005. *Chutu wangyi gu yiji yanjiu* 出土亡佚古醫籍研究. Beijing: Zhongyi guji chubanshe.

1990. *Zhongyi wenxian xue* 中醫文獻學. Shanghai: Shanghai kexue jishu.

Masuzawa, Tomoko. 2005. *The Invention of World Religions: Or, How European Universalism Was Preserved in the Language of Pluralism*. Chicago: University of Chicago Press.

McLeod, Katrina, and Robin D. S. Yates. 1981. "Forms of Ch'in Law: An Annotated Translation of the *Feng-chen shih*." *Harvard Journal of Asiatic Studies* 41.1: 111–63.

Mueggler, Erik. 2011. *The Paper Road: Archive and Experience in the Botanical Exploration of Western China and Tibet*. Berkeley: University of California Press.

Needham, Joseph. 1974. *Science and Civilisation in China, Vol. 5, Chemistry and Chemical Technology, Part 2, Spagyrical Discovery and Invention: Magisteries of Gold and Immortality*. Cambridge: Cambridge University Press.

Needham, Joseph, and Lu Gwei-djen. 2000. Rpt. 2004. *Science and Civilisation, Volume 6, Part 6, Biology and Biological Technology: Medicine*, edited by Nathan Sivin. Cambridge: Cambridge University Press.

Ngo Van Xuyet. 1976. *Divination, magie et politique dans la Chine ancienne: essai.* Paris: Presses universitaires de France.

Nutton, Vivian. 2004. *Ancient Medicine.* Abingdon: Routledge.

Nylan, Michael. 2011. *Yang Xiong and the Pleasures of Reading and Classical Learning in China.* New Haven, CT: American Oriental Society.

2009. "Classics without Canonization: Reflections on Classical Learning and Authority in Qin (221–210 BC) and Han (206 BC–AD 220)." In *Early Chinese Religion, Part One, Shang through Han (1250 BC–AD 220)*, edited by John Lagerwey and Marc Kalinowski, I: 721–76. Leiden, The Netherlands: Brill.

2007 [2005–2006]. "Notes on a Case of Illicit Sex from Zhangjiashan: A Translation and Commentary." *Early China* 30: 25–45.

2000. "Textual Authority in Pre-Han and Han." *Early China* 25: 205–58.

Okanishi Tameto 岡西為人. 1977. *Song yiqian yiji kao* 宋以前醫籍考. Taipei: Nantian shuju.

Peabody, Norbert. 2001. "Cents, Sense, Census: Human Inventories in Late Precolonial and Early Colonial India." *Comparative Studies of Society and History* 43.4: 819–50.

Peng Jinhua 彭錦華. 1999. "Guanju Qin Han mu qingli jianbao" 關沮秦漢墓清理簡報. *Wenwu* 文物 1999.6: 26–47.

Petersen, Jens Østergård. 1995. "Which Books Did the First Emperor of Ch'in Burn? On the Meaning of 'Pai Chia' in Early Chinese Sources." *Monumenta Serica* 43: 1–52.

Pines, Yuri. 2002. *Foundations of Confucian Thought: Intellectual Life in the Chunqiu Period, 722–453 B.C.E.* Honolulu: University of Hawaii Press.

Pollack, Sheldon. 2009. "Future Philology? The Fate of a Soft Science in a Hard World." *Critical Inquiry* 35.4: 931–61.

Porkert, Mansvelt. 1974. *The Theoretical Foundations of Chinese Medicine: Systems of Correspondence.* Boston: MIT Press.

Qian Chaochen 錢超塵. 2010. "Songben 'Shanghanlun' banben jiankao" 宋本《傷寒論》版本簡考. *Henan zhongyi* 河南中醫 2010.1: 1–9.

1993. *Shanghan lun wenxian tongkao* 傷寒論文獻通考. Beijing: Xueyuan chubanshe.

1983. "Kangzhi ben 'Shanghan lun' kao" 《康治本傷寒論》考. *Beijing zhongyi zazhi* 北京中醫雜志 1983.3: 45–47.

Qian Yuzhi 錢玉趾. 2014. "Xin faxian Bi Xi yilun de bianxi" 新發現 《蔽昔醫論》的辨析. *Wenshi zazhi* 文史雜志 2014.2: 24.

Raphals, Lisa. 1998. *Sharing the Light: Representations of Women and Virtue in Early China.* Albany: State University of New York Press.

Rogaski, Ruth. 2004. *Hygienic Modernity: Meanings of Health and Disease in Treaty-Port China.* Berkeley: University of California Press.

Salguero, Pierce. 2009. "The Buddhist Medicine King in Literary Context: Reconsidering an Early Medieval Example of Indian Influence on Chinese Medicine and Surgery." *History of Religions* 48.3: 183–210.

Sanft, Charles. 2013. "Qin Government: Structures, Principles, and Practices." In *Qin – the Eternal Emperor and His Terracotta Warriors*, edited by Maria Khayutina. 118–29. Zürich: Neue Zürcher Zeitung Libro.

2005a. "Rule: A Study of Jia Yi's *Xinshu*." Inaugural diss., University of Müenster.

2005b. "Six of One, Two Dozen of the Other: The Abatement of Mutilating Punishments under Han Emperor Wen." *Asia Major*, 3rd Series 18.1: 79–100.

Schaberg, David. 2001. *A Patterned Past: Form and Thought in Early Chinese Historiography*. Cambridge, MA: Harvard University Asia Center.

Scheid, Volker. 2012. "Defining the Best Practice or Cultivating the Best Practitioners." In *Integrating East Asian Medicine into Contemporary Healthcare*, edited by Volker Scheid and Hugh MacPherson, 13–37. Edinburgh: Churchill Livingstone.

2008. "Globalizing Chinese Medical Understandings of Menopause." *East Asian Science and Technology* 2: 485–506.

2007. *Currents of Tradition in Chinese Medicine, 1626–2006*. Seattle: Eastland Press.

2002. *Chinese Medicine in Contemporary China: Plurality and Synthesis*. Durham, NC: Duke University Press.

2001. "Shaping Chinese Medicine: Two Case Studies from Contemporary China." In *Innovation in Chinese Medicine*, edited by Elisabeth Hsu, 370–404. Cambridge: Cambridge University Press.

Shapin, Steven. 2010. *Never Pure: Historical Studies of Science as If It Was Produced by People with Bodies, Situated in Time, Space, Culture, and Society, and Struggling for Credibility and Authority*. Baltimore: Johns Hopkins University Press.

Shen Pei 沈培. 2007. "Cong Zhanguo jian kan guren zhanbu de bizhi – jianlun yisui shuo 從戰國簡看古人占卜的"蔽志– 兼論「移祟」說." *Guwen zi yu gudai shi* 1 古文字與古代史: 391–434.

Shinno, Reiko. 2007. "Medical Schools and the Temples of the Three Progenitors in Yuan China: A Case of Cross-Cultural Interactions." *Harvard Journal of Asiatic Studies* 67.1: 89–133.

Sivin, Nathan. Forthcoming. *Healthcare in Eleventh-Century China.*

2012. "Therapy and Antiquity in Late Imperial China." In *Antiquarianism and Intellectual Life in Europe and China, 1500–1800*, edited by Peter N. Miller and François Louis, 222–33. Ann Arbor: University of Michigan Press.

2007. "Foreword." In *Currents of Tradition in Chinese Medicine, 1626–2006*, by Volker Scheid, xv–xvii. Seattle: Eastland Press.

2000. "Editor's Introduction." In *Science and Civilisation, Volume 6, Part 6, Biology and Biological Technology: Medicine*, by Joseph Needham and Lu Gwei-djen, edited by Nathan Sivin, 1–37. Cambridge: Cambridge University Press.

1995. "Text and Experience in Classical Chinese Medicine." In *Knowledge and the Scholarly Medical Traditions, edited by Don Bates*, 177–204. Cambridge: Cambridge University Press.

1993. "*Huang ti nei ching.*" In *Early Chinese Texts: A Bibliographical Guide*, edited by Michael Loewe, 196–215. Berkeley: Society for the Study of Early China.

1978. *Traditional Medicine in Contemporary China: A Partial Translation of Revised Outline of Chinese Medicine (1972) with an Introductory Study on Change in Present-Day and Early Medicine.* Ann Arbor: University of Michigan, Center for Chinese Studies.

1968. *Chinese Alchemy: Preliminary Studies.* Cambridge, MA: Harvard University Press.

Smith, Kidder. 1989. "*Zhouyi* Interpretation from Accounts in the *Zuozhuan*." *Harvard Journal of Asiatic Studies* 49.2: 421–63.

Standaert, Nicolas. 1999. "The Jesuits Did NOT Manufacture 'Confucianism.'" *East Asian Science, Technology, Medicine* 16: 115–32.

Sun, Anna Xiao Dong. 2013. *Confucianism as a World Religion: Contested Histories and Contemporary Realities.* Princeton, NJ: Princeton University Press.

Taniguchi Hiroshi 谷口洋. 2010. "Fu ni jijo o tsukeru koto: Ryō Kan no majiwari ni okeru sakusha no mezame" 賦に自序をつけること：兩漢の交における作者のめざめ. *Tōhōgaku* 東方學 119: 22–39.

Taylor, Kim. 2005. *Chinese Medicine in Early Communist China, 1945–1963: A Medicine of Revolution.* London and New York: RoutledgeCurzon.

Temkin, Owsei. 1991. *Hippocrates in a World of Pagans and Christians.* Baltimore: Johns Hopkins University Press.

Trautmann, Thomas. 2011. "The Past in the Present." *Fragments: Interdisciplinary Approaches to the Study of Ancient and Medieval Pasts* 1: 2–20.

2006. *Languages and Nations: The Dravidian Proof in Colonial Madras.* Berkeley: University of California Press.

1997. Rpt. 2008. *Aryans and British India.* New Delhi: Yoda Press.

Tsien, Tsuen-hsuin. 2004. *Written on Bamboo and Silk: The Beginnings of Chinese Books and Inscriptions, 2nd ed.* Chicago: University of Chicago Press.

1985. *Science and Civilisation in China: Volume 5, Chemistry and Chemical Technology; Part 1, Paper and Printing.* Cambridge: Cambridge University Press.

Twitchett, Denis, and Michael Loewe, eds. 1986. *The Cambridge History of China: Volume I: The Ch'in and Han Empires, 221 B.C.–A.D. 220.* Cambridge: Cambridge University Press.

Unschuld, Paul. 2003. *Huang di nei jing su wen: Nature: Knowledge, Imagery in an Ancient Chinese Medical Text.* Berkeley: University of California Press.

1986. *Nan-ching: The Classic of Difficult Issues.* Berkeley: University of California Press.

Wagner, Robert G. 1973. "Lebenstil und Drogen im chinesischen Mittelalter." *T'oung Pao* 59: 79–178.

Wagoner, Philip B. 2003. "Precolonial Intellectuals and the Production of Colonial Knowledge." *Comparative Studies of Society and History* 45.4: 783–814.

Wang Aihe. 2000. *Cosmology and Political Culture in Early China.* Cambridge: Cambridge University Press.

Wang Jimin 王吉民. 1930. *Zhongguo lidai yixue zhi faming* 中國歷代醫學之發明. Shanghai: Xinzhong yishe.

Wang Pinxian 王聘賢, Ding Qihou 丁啟後, and Zhou Hongjin 周洪進. 1982. "Shanghan lun zixu kaoping" 《傷寒論》自序考評. *Yunnan zhongyi xueyuan xuebao* 雲南中醫學院學報 1982.4: 23–4.

Wang Yong 王勇, and Gao Ailing 高愛玲. 2006. "Wang ben he Zhao ben Zhujie shanghan lun bijiao" 汪本和趙本《注解傷寒論》比較. *Zhongyi wenxian zazhi* 中醫文獻杂志 2006.4: 4–8.

Winchester, Simon. 2008. *The Man Who Loved China: The Fantastic Story of the Eccentric Scientist Who Unlocked the Mysteries of the Middle Kingdom*. New York: HarperCollins.

Wong K. Chimin [Wang Jimin], and Wu Lien-teh. 1932. *History of Chinese Medicine: Being a Chronicle of Medical Happenings in China from Ancient Times to the Present Period*. Tientsin: Tientsin Press.

Wu Chengluo 吳承洛. 1957. *Zhongguo duliang hengshi* 中國度量衡史. Shanghai: Shangwu yinshuguan.

Wu Lien-teh. 1959. *Plague Fighter: The Autobiography of a Modern Chinese Physician*. Cambridge: W. Hefer & Sons.

Wu, Yi-Li. 2013. "The Qing Period." In *Chinese Medicine and Healing: An Illustrated History*, edited by T. J. Hinrichs and Linda L. Barnes, 161–207. Cambridge, MA: Belknap Press of Harvard University Press.

Wu Yiyi. 1994. "A Medical Line of Many Masters: A Prosopographical Study of Liu Wansu and His Disciples from the Jin to the Early Ming." *Chinese Science* 11: 36–65.

Xie Guihua. 2005. "Han Bamboo and Wooden Medical Records Discovered in Military Sites from the North-Western Frontier Regions." In *Medieval Chinese Medicine: The Dunhuang Medical Manuscripts*, edited by Christopher Cullen and Vivienne Lo, 77–106. London: RoutledgeCurzon.

Xing Wen. 2013. "The Hexagram Gu." In *Chinese Medicine and Healing: An Illustrated History*, edited by T. J. Hinrichs and Linda L. Barnes, 20–1. Cambridge, MA: Belknap Press of Harvard University Press.

Yamada Keiji 山田慶兒. 2003. *Zhongguo gudai yixue de xingcheng* 中國古代醫學的形成. Translated by Liao Yuqun 廖育群 and Li Jianmin 李建民. Taipei: Dongda tushu gongsi.

1998. *The Origins of Acupuncture, Moxibustion, and Decoction*. Kyoto: International Research Center for Japanese Studies.

1990. *Yoru naku tori: igaku, jujutsu, densetsu* 夜鳴く鳥: 医学・呪術・伝説. Tokyo: Iwanami Shoten.

1988. "Henjaku densetsu" 扁鵲傳說. *Tōhō gakuhō* 東方學報 60: 73–158.

1985. *Shinhatsugen Chūgoku kagakushi shiryō no kenkyū* 新發現中國科學史資料の研究. Kyoto: Kyōto Daigaku Jinbun Kagaku Kenkyūjo.

Yan Shiyun 嚴世蕓. 1990. *Zhongguo yiji tongkao* 中國醫籍通考. Shanghai: Shanghai zhongyi xueyuan.

Yao Chunpeng 姚春鵬. 2008. *Huangdi neijing – Qi guannian xia de tianren yixue* 黃帝內經-氣觀念下的天人醫學. Beijing: Zhonghua shuju.

Ye Fazheng 葉發正. 1995. *Shanghan xueshu shi* 傷寒學術史. Hubei: Huazhong shifan daxue chubanshe.

Yu Jiaxi 余嘉錫. 1997. *Yu Jiaxi wenshi lunji* 余嘉錫文史論集. Changsha: Yuelu shushe.

1985. *Gushu tongli* 古書通例. Shanghai: Shanghai guji.

Zhan, Mei. 2009. *Other-worldly: Making Chinese Medicine through Transnational Frames*. Durham, NC: Duke University Press.

Zhang Canjia 张灿玾. 1998. *Zhongyi guji wenxian xue* 中醫古籍文獻學. Beijing: Renmin weisheng.

Zhang Taiyan 章太炎. 1982 [1986]. *Zhang Taiyan quanji* 章太炎全集. Vol. 5. Shanghai: Shanghai renmin chubanshe.

Zhao Hongjun 趙洪鈞. 1989. *Jindai Zhongxiyao lunzheng shi* 近代中西醫論爭史. Hefei: Anhui kexue jishu.

Zheng Jinsheng 鄭金生, and Li Jianmin 李建民. 1997. "Xiandai Zhongguo yixueshi yanjiu de yuanliu" 現代中國醫學史研究的源流. *Dalu zazhi* 大陸雜志 95.6: 266–74.

Zhou Lisheng 周立升, and Wang Demin 王德敏. 1989. *Chunqiu zhexue* 春秋哲學. N.p.: Shandong daxue chubanshe.

Zhou Yimou 周一謀. 1994. *Mawangdui yixue wenhua* 馬王堆醫學文化. Shanghai: Wenhui.

Zhu Diguang 朱迪光. 1985. "Lun Hou Hanshu Zhang Zhongjing zhi wu zhuan: Shijie Jiyidongdong zhi yi" 論後漢書張仲景之無傳:試解吉益東洞之疑. In *Zhongguo zhongyi yanjiuyuan sanshinian lunwenxuan* 中國中醫研究院三十年論文選 *(1955–1985)*, ed. Zhongguo zhongyi yanjiuyuan 中國中醫研究院. 451–4. Beijing: Zhongguo guji.

Zhu Jianping 朱建平. 2003. *Zhongguo yixue shi yanjiu* 中國醫學史研究. Beijing: Zhongyi guji chubanshe.

INDEX